Whole Person Healing

The O-Ring Imaging Technique:
Influences to Oriental and Occidental Medicine

By Phillip Shinnick, Ph. D., L. Ac., and
Adriano Borgna, M.D. L. Ac.

AuthorHouse™
1663 Liberty Drive, Suite 200
Bloomington, IN 47403
www.authorhouse.com
Phone: 1-800-839-8640

First published by AuthorHouse 11/25/2009

ISBN: 978-1-4389-6566-6 (sc)

Library of Congress Control Number: 2009902979

Printed in the United States of America
Bloomington, Indiana

This book is printed on acid-free paper.

authorHOUSE®

ACKNOWLEDGEMENTS:

The following individuals have contributed to this work. Celia Blumenthal, M.D., Herbert Berger, OBT., the physicians and therapists at the Center for Dance and Sport Medicine in Manhattan from 1984-1990, BJ Cling, Ph.D., J.D., Roberta Flack, Patrick LaRiccia, M.D., M. Sc., M.A., Catherine Gehm, Laurence Porter, Xiao Yan, Carol Karlson, Rustum Roy, Ph.D., Jack Haddad, M.D., M.B.A., Garry Williams, Richard Malter, Neri Kedem, Larry Tan, John Pinto, Donna De Verona and Guy Obolensky.

TABLE OF CONTENTS

INTRODUCTION

In science we like data, especially through time, with the same technique. We had this situation with Yoshiaki Omura, a Japanese/American medical doctor (M.D.), an electrical engineer, a Doctor of Science (Sc. D. Columbia Medical School), a publisher in Traditional Chinese Medicine, an editor of a major International Journal, has published numerous articles for twenty five years using a no cost diagnostic tool, based upon finger strength, which has original data. The medical establishment likes very expensive technical sophisticated equipment, so does not much notice his work; there is really no money in it. Real scientists are very interested. He has photographed all of his results and does an exhaustive intake of each patient. Sometimes it takes him up to eight hours. He is a real scientist, exposing everything he does to scrutiny by keeping meticulous records.

Yet here we have data, right before our eyes with confounding results, a mark of a good scientist, to report all results, no matter how contradictory to medical or scientific understandings. Parts of his work have been confirmed by others, over the years, for example, the existence of bacteria in the stomach leading to ulcers (some Australian scientist got the Nobel Prize for this) and he mapped the migration of bacteria from the stomach to the heart causing a confounding result which could not be helped with heart medication. He found the type of bacteria and matched the right antibiotic to it and got good results.

His analysis of Traditional Chinese Medicine, based upon results of his O-Ring Test, is remarkable; yet who understands all these angles: science, electro-magnetism, and Oriental and Occidental medicine? We needed an interpreter, so I called Phil Shinnick, who worked with Omura for eight years, as his right hand man, Secretary of his college and an Editor of his Journal. They haven't worked together for the last fifteen years; a good prospect to get an unbiased analysis for what the O-ring is all about. I wanted to know, what is this finger business? So many articles, and each one almost one hundred pages, he doesn't mess around, he put it all out there, but it is too much to absorb or understand.

Phil Shinnick himself strides many fields, an Olympian and World Record holder in the long jump, a Ph.D. from UC Berkeley, an Assistant Professor at Rutgers, and Assistant Clinical Professor at New York Medical College. He now has a small subsidy from a privately endowed research fund.

So I asked Shinnick if he could write a book about the O-Ring Test. He was the only one I knew who had read most of Omura's work and assisted in many key experiments. He himself has a clinical practice in acupuncture with a New York acupuncture license. He also publishes in Gaussian (magnetic) and columbic (electric) energy fields, heart disease, and Qigong. He has written for the New York Times and other popular publications. I asked him to present his scientific research at several of the Whole Person Healing conferences, which I coordinated.

Really a thankless job, but what I had in mind was answering some important questions. Is this good for people? Does it assist in healing? Is it practical and does anyone do it today in the world? Are there any good scientific results? What about contributions to Oriental or Occidental Medicine? How do you do this O-ring test? Shinnick has already published on the technique in the American Journal of Acupuncture, and some research on the O-ring in Medical Acupuncture, a physicians/acupuncturist journal. We needed more.

In this book he summarizes Omura's early work and lists the contributions to medicine and science and tries to explain the significance to healing. It is far too much to list in this introduction, but it suffices to say Omura has made contributions to traditional and modern medicine. He has been able to image internal organs on the surface of the body and map the pathways of these organs and compare these images to traditional understandings. He has been able to map the migration of microorganisms in the body and expand on the understanding of traditional medicine. He has done scientific experiments to see what is behind the O-ring.

Well, it was about seven years ago that I asked Shinnick to help me bring Omura's O-ring to light and it has been difficult. So he recruited some help along the way. He asked Adriano Borgna, M.D. L.Ac., who teaches at the Pacific School of Acupuncture in New York, to cover medical aspects of healing. He has attended Omura physician training programs for certification of physician acupuncturists since 1985 and is a highly respected student of Omura. Borgna helped Shinnick systematically go through all of Omura's O-ring articles up to about ten years ago. He and Shinnick also put together a chart showing all the front and back points for organs used in diagnosis. Shinnick has been the engine behind this.

I then asked Shinnick if he knew anyone who actually used the O-ring in clinical practice and if this technique was helping people in healing. Two practitioners who had read his research in journals contacted him, Richard Malter from Australia and Neri Kedem from Israel. Shinnick named both men research assistants under his Research Institute of Global Physiology, Behavior and Treatment, Inc. I gave them a grant to travel to our Whole Person Healing Conferences to see what they were up to, and they did not disappoint us. Omura was skeptical. He put them through the ringer, not giving them much of a role in his yearly Symposium, but they stuck with it and learned how to write a scientific paper and he called them front and center to deliver a paper on studies and techniques they were using. So each appears in this book explaining the contributions they have made to Oriental and Occidental medicine, and how they have helped people. Now it seems they are within the Omura fold. They are not physicians but earnest young healers who have training in Oriental medicine techniques but have also learned how to talk science, write articles and heal people using the O-ring. They are regulars at Omura's teachings.

As for Shinnick, he did a seven-year study using the O-ring and another ten years figuring out what he had on his hands. Like Omura he photographed all results. He had physicians independently evaluate clinical study patients and did a standard protocol for each. He then tries to offer a theory of the O-ring, which he calls the Hui hypothesis, based on his imagings and samples of Omura's imagings. In short, it appears that there exist rings near what has been described by ancients as acupuncture points, but Shinnick and Omura have found these to be large and change size according to stimulation by acupuncture, Qigong, or manual or electrical stimulation. Shinnick hypothesizes that these circles are in constant flux and the O-ring catches them in a dominant phase, which differs according to the patient and problem. For the lung and heart there are numerous phases and people get stuck in a certain phase manifest in certain patterns. Shinnick finds some differences between the lung and colon in traditional theory and images ovary pathways never before done. Omura finds more pathways for the stomach pathway. Malter and Kedem each find new things in traditional theory, which is useful for patients, primarily in organ relationships to each other.

Outsiders sometimes think that scientists are all rationalists, but in natural philosophy, under which material science and medicine are subheads, we also listen to our minds. Shinnick paints pictures of what his mind thinks about the data he is confronted with. These paintings are used as theoretical references to phase changes that are seen with the data and experimentation. Art and science are not far apart. We need to be creative if we are going to get very far with nature and phenomenon. Creation is stretched all over the place and we are all a part of it.

There will be others, I hope, through this work who will be able to test medicines especially in places where there is limited access to medicines or advice from pharmacologists. For a scientist using this method, speculations could be tested at no cost and results could lead to more confidence in following a certain direction. Healers can test weakness in the body, organ dysfunction, circulation problems, evaluating the results of treatment, the presence of micro-organisms and herbal, medicinal or nutritional additives which might help in healing.

Rustum Roy

Member American, Japanese, English and Indian Academies of Science

Eugene Pugh Professor Emeritus of the Solid State,
Pennsylvania State University
Distinguished Professor of Materials, Arizona State University Visiting Professor of Medicine,
University of Arizona Chair, Friends of Health

CHAPTER ONE
DISCOVERY AND DEVELOPMENT

BACKGROUND

In the late 1970s Dr. Yoshiaki Omura — physician, engineer, researcher and author — was testing arm strength using applied kinesiology when he felt that there must be a better and easier method to determine arm strength. In the process he discovered the Bi-digital-O-ring test, a sensitive, non-invasive diagnostic screening method that can provide basic information about a variety of pathologies. This test, also known as the ORT, BDORT or Omura O-ring, is now taught at two schools in Japan and accepted by the western medical community. It can be used in acupuncture, dentistry, and veterinary medicine.

The ORT has many advantages. It is quick, safe and low-cost, and there is no expensive equipment to maintain — an important point in this era of ever-rising medical costs. Easily administered, it can discriminate between normal and abnormal tissue and, as a primary screening method, it can provide important information to health practitioners without exposing patients to more expensive and invasive procedures such as MRIs, CT scans, X-rays or exploratory surgery and the ancillary concerns about strong magnetic fields and radiation as well as surgical recovery.

In this book we will describe this easy to learn procedure and delve into its history and development and discuss the enormous implications of its application in almost every aspect of science and medicine as well as its role in healing and self-care. In later chapters we will talk about its uses in daily life, e.g. how to determine an individual's appropriate nutritional needs or their body's reaction to drugs and dosages. Clinical experiences will be explored and suggestions for ordinary application will be offered. In many cases just an understanding of a particular reaction is enough to influence behavior. Other chapters will show how, sometimes, this procedure can offer a new interpretation of traditional understanding in Chinese Medicine and its hypothesis. And while Dr. Omura made many observations from the O-ring experiments, only a few of them will be explored in this book.

Sometimes the ORT, when used in the imaging of the internal organ pathways and meridians on the skin, generates new and sometimes conflicting findings when compared with those of traditional Chinese Medicine, as will be shown in the subsequent chapters.

From 1984-1990 Dr. Shinnick worked as a researcher with Dr. Omura and was present for most of the scientific and clinical research he did. During that time Dr. Shinnick also edited, wrote and organized international scientific symposia with Dr. Omura for the journal, *Acupuncture and Electro-therapeutics Research,* the *International Journal* – the organ of the International College of

Acupuncture and Electro-therapeutics. At that time Dr. Shinnick co-authored an historical article on Oriental and Occidental pulse diagnosis in the 15th to 18th centuries and published a public learning monograph on the heart for The Heart Disease Research Foundation along with several other authors.[1,2] Since then he has worked independently on this test and published a guide to using the ORT in its clinical application on toxic organ pathways in the *Journal of American Acupuncture* and in *Medical Acupuncture.* [3,4] Additionally, electrical engineer Michael Losco published a synopsis of the method, including some procedures and capabilities of the test.[5]

Dr. Adriano Borgna, co-author of this book, is an Italian physician, a licensed acupuncturist in NY State and a faculty member of the Pacific College of Oriental Medicine who attended medical acupuncture training courses taught by Dr. Omura at the International College of Acupuncture and Electro-therapeutics, which was headed by Dr. Omura from 1988-1992. Since that time he has periodically attended additional physician training seminars at the school.

In this book we will summarize Dr. Omura's scientific research and clinical cases using the ORT that he has presented in his Journal and lectures and taught in his physician-training courses for twenty-five years. In addition to frequent journal articles chronicling his observations regarding the O-ring in English, Dr. Omura has published two books in Spanish and one in Japanese. [6,7]

Yoshiaki Omura trained as a physician (MD), and electrical engineer (MS), did a surgical on-cology residency at Columbia Medical School and advanced work in pharmacology and electric-physiology (Sc.D.). He was the first to measure the potential of a single cardiac cell. Later on he became a Heart Disease Research director, and author of a book on Traditional Chinese Medicine. [8, 8a] He is also President of the International College of Acupuncture and Electro-therapeutics and editor of the school's International Journal. His training and knowledge are manifest in his 25 years of research that started with the investigation of Applied-Kinesiology and ended with the discovery of the ORT or O-ring Test (Bi-Digital-O-Ring Test) and its innumerable applications. He criticized the traditional arm pull method by showing unreliability in arm strength, fatigue from changes in brain circulation, and a time-bound ghost effect from each attempt.

DISCOVERY AND DEVELOPMENT

Dr. Omura discovered the ORT while he was testing the grasping strength of a hand that was being subjected to battery-generated positive and negative electro-magnetic fields in close proximity to the subject. Both positive and negative fields were shown to have an effect on the grasping strength of the hand and finger, along with various sounds and whether the subject's eyes were open or closed. [9, 10, 11, 12]

He then confirmed the O-ring phenomenon while investigating pain threshold and grip force in relationship to brain laterality. He noticed that when applying pressure to create pain, the grip force decreased. He observed that (a) induced pain would decrease the grip force, and (b) even a light pressure on skin areas, very often related to "previous pain," also reproduced this phenomenon. However, pressure applied on "normal" areas did not cause the grip force to decrease. [13, 14, 15]

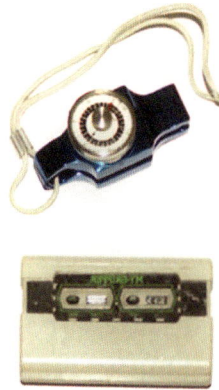

Figure 1 (Top: Thumb and Finger Strength Meter)
(Bottom: Hand Grip Force meter)

Subsequently, Omura also noticed that, rather than using full-hand grip force, it was also possible to utilize a subject's resistance to having the thumb and one finger of the same hand pried apart from one another when held "tip-to-tip," thus forming the characteristic "O-ring" position for which the method is named. The relative strength of the response was noted.

Through trial and error, he was able to elucidate conditions under which the O-ring resistance yielded confirmation of a known pathology and its exact boundaries. The accumulation of this information lent support to the possibility that it involved an electro-magnetic phenomenon, specifically a *resonance phenomenon.* (See Chapter 2: Theory)

In continued investigations, [16, 17, 18, 19] Omura showed that the ORT could be used as a research and pre-screening tool before administering standard Western diagnostic tests, thus providing a reliable guide for treatment. He also demonstrated its utility for compatibility testing of food and drugs, as well as their toxicity and dosage. Additionally, he noted that its usefulness was not limited to Western medical applications. In Chapter Six there is a detailed case of a breast cancer patient and the testing substances beneficial against that particular cancer as examined by Dr. Omura and Shinnick, and in Chapter Seven Shinnick shows adverse reactions to the gall bladder from alcohol and food to the hip area.

A series of experiments led to the concept of electro-magnetic field resonance as the scientific understanding behind the ORT. The initial presentation relates the technique, history, development and application by Omura to various clinical cases. The purpose of this book is to provide an independent analysis of the O-ring test and its application to healing and ordinary uses by practitioners and individuals.

METHOD

Using the ORT with the proper control substance held in a subject's hand, one can stimulate the surface of the subject's skin with an insulated probe and get either a positive or negative response from that location as to whether there is a resonance between the control substance and that particular spot. (Figure 2A, 2B, 2C, and 3) This will translate into a decreased muscular strength that manifests in the weakening of the ring that is formed when the tip of the subject's thumb touches the tip of any other finger of the same hand. The control substance can be any microorganism such as a virus, bacteria, parasite, fungus, a sample of an organ, any other cellular sample (in the form of microscopic slide, or pure sample), heavy or light metal, a drug or a supplement, a neurotransmitter or a tumor marker. It can include a tissue sample of different organs such as the heart, stomach or liver, and a sample of a biochemical present in either a normal or abnormal functioning organ (see below 4A, 4B). [20, 21, 22, 23]

With the discovery of the indirect method, (see Chapter 3, Materials and Methods) using a third person to test a subject, Dr. Omura was able to test almost anything that needed to be tested, from paraplegic patients to children, and from animals to cadavers. (Figure 3) Briefly, instead of an insulated probe touching the surface of the subject, the third person holds an electrical conducting probe in his or her hand while stimulating the subject.

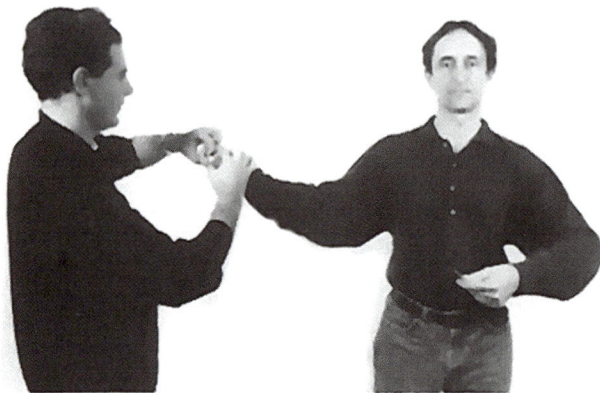

Direct Approach
Figure 2A
Closed position with a non-conductive probe in subject's hand

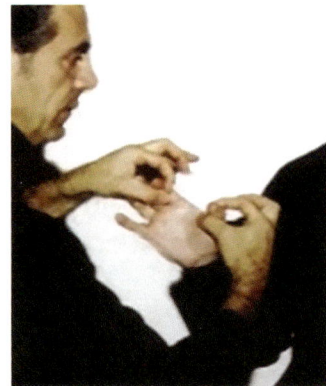

2B
Finger open position

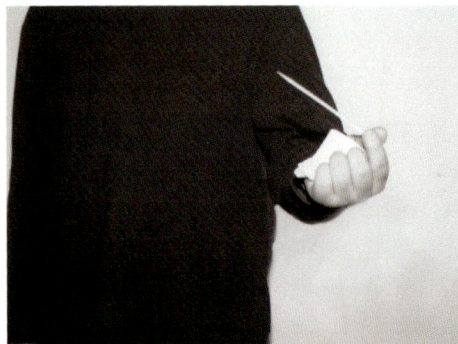

Figure 2C
Control reference substance in a piece of paper
with a non-conducting probe.

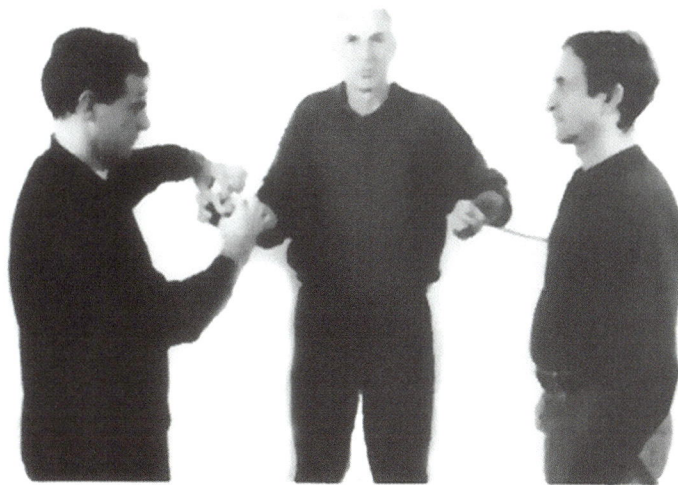

Figure 3
Indirect O-ring Test in a closed position holding a conducting probe

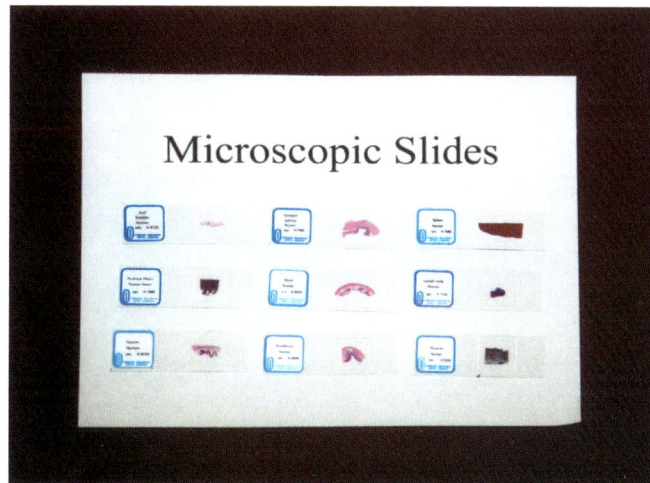

Figure 4A
Top of picture: Herpes Virus, Hg, TromboxanB2,
Acetylcholine, Integrin Oncogene fos
Bottom of picture: O-ring Probes (For Direct & Indirect)

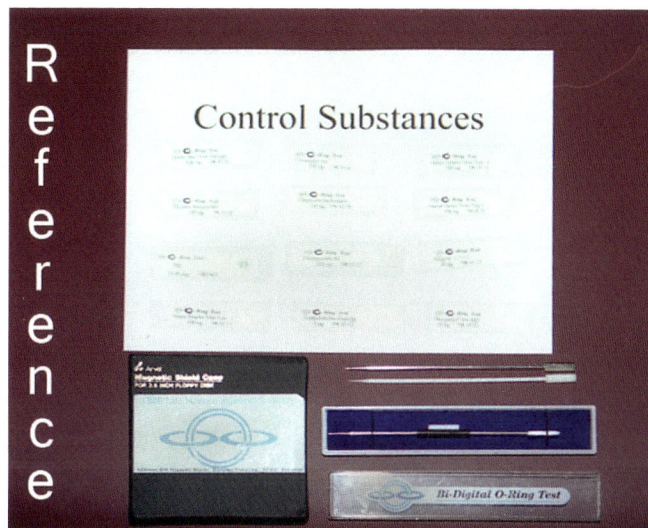

Figure 4B Microscopic Samples

Dr. Omura suspected that the information of the electro-magnetic field responsible for the ORT could be transported at a distance and started experimenting with a photon-generated laser (8mm-wat) with a monochromatic concentrated beam. He focused the laser on the organ representation point of the stomach (中脘ZhongWan) from a distance of about twenty feet after putting a known toxin to the stomach (aspirin) in the hand of the subject, and he then recorded a weakening of the O-ring. Next, he put the aspirin in the vicinity of the laser beam and recorded a weakening of the O-ring in the subject holding the laser pointer (third person indirect method). In other words, he was able to test a subject at a distance using the laser beam as the probe in the indirect method. This demonstrated that the information of the electro-magnetic field, in this case, the aspirin and the stomach, could be carried at a distance. It had to be bi-directional to evoke a response in the third person. Consequently, this led to other experiments with X-rays, CT -scans, MRIs, electron microscopes, and magnification of those images reflected onto a larger field such as a screen. [24] An individual can experiment with control substances to find out about the presence of a virus, parasite, bacteria, toxin or heavy metal that may be in the body on any of the above procedures.

If a photon-generated laser could be a means of bi-directional communication then could this happen with an organ meridian pathway on the body, since the organ generates energy? Was there an organ-generated, concentrated electro-magnetic field with information on that pathway known as meridians? Was there a correspondence between the organ-generated energy and the *umunculus* (from Latin: little man) found in the ear, hand, foot etc…? These were the questions and Dr. Omura's experiments and publications helped answer most of them. (Figure 6 See later chapter on Traditional Chinese Medicine)

Generally speaking, Omura has found that, the greater the experience of the examiner with the use of the O-ring test, and the more time devoted to the testing process with each subject, the more comprehensive the results will be. Thereby, the sophistication and interpretation of the results of the O-ring test will be commensurate with an individual's understanding of their field of medicine and science; likewise, for someone in the field of complementary medicine, such as Oriental medicine, acupuncture, herbology or homeopathy. According to the research and observations of Losco, "… the O-ring test has frequently succeeded in identifying patients' problems where expensive laboratory equipment and procedures have failed. The O-ring test is presently being used by many physicians around the world and it is being taught in some medical schools in Japan, Finland and Venezuela." [5(p54)]

Since 1995 an International Symposium on ORT has been held in Japan and there are two schools in Tokyo that teach ORT just to medical doctors.

CHAPTER TWO
THEORY OF THE O-RING TEST PHENOMENON AND EXPERIMENTAL EVIDENCE TO SUPPORT IT

Dr. Omura postulated that the mechanism of the O-ring response may be due to a resonance phenomenon between two substances having an identical electro-magnetic wave frequency separated by a distance. [25(p128)] Conditions, which support this theory, are as follows.

a). The O-ring test may fail if performed in close proximity to a source of an electro-magnetic field, such as a transformer or solenoid, or the running motor of an electric fan, refrigerator or other electronic equipment. (The signal travels in a field perpendicular to the flow of electrons or photons. Electro-magnetic background noise would also interrupt such a signal. [19])

b). The O-ring may fail if a person is electrically grounded, e.g., stands barefoot on a damp floor, or physically touches an electrical ground such as radiator, faucet or grounded electric appliance.

c). The O-ring test may fail if the patient or examiner is wearing a metal watchband, bracelet or necklace. These metal objects that encircle the arm or neck will interfere with the electro-magnetic signal traveling along the arm to the brain.

d). The O-ring test fails to identify a food or medicine that is enclosed in a metal container or wrapped in metal foil.

e). The O-ring test may become inaccurate if the patient uses his own free finger or a metal rod to touch his own bare skin. This is similar to an electrical short circuit, and the signal bypasses the brain. During the O-ring test, when the patient touches his own body, he should use only a non-metallic substance such as a plastic or wooden stick.

f). The electro-magnetic nature of the O-ring test is further demonstrated during the indirect method of testing in which a metal conductor is used.

Omura also showed that the polarity of a field interrupts the O-ring test, as it does for electro-magnetism. [19]

One of the most convincing explanations on the physiologic mechanism involved in the ORT has been the one that Dr. Chifuyu Takeshige (former Dean & Chairman of the 1ˢᵗ Dept. of Physiology, Showa University School of Medicine) first postulated in 1994 and then confirmed in 1997 during the International Symposium on ORT in Tokyo. According to this theory the pineal gland is the sensor responsible for the detection of the resonance phenomenon when two identical substances are present; one inside the body, and the other one in contact or close proximity to the body.

Dr. Takeshige had observed that the ORT was not reliable in a patient with a tumor of the pineal gland. It was also determined that the ORT is not reliable if the subject has his/her eyes closed (the pineal gland is sensitive to light), or if the subject is exposed to a magnetic field because it inhibits the enzyme that converts serotonin to N-*Acetylserotonin* [NAT] in the pineal gland.

The voluntary muscle contraction in the ORT is performed by the α-motor-neuron and the γ-motor-neuron. The latter is activated by the descending serotonergic system originating in the *raphé nucleus* in the brainstem. Since the *raphé nucleus* is activated by serotonin, the muscle tone changes according to the amount of serotonin released in the brain. The concentration of serotonin in the pineal gland is 50-100 times higher than in the brainstem.

According to Dr. Takeshige there are two kinds of cells in the pineal gland, one that responds to magnetic fields and another that responds to light. The latter seems to be the sensor that might explain the phenomena observed in the ORT by inhibition of the NAT enzymatic activity. This, in turn, changes the amount of serotonin released, therefore influencing the descending fibers of the γ-motor-neuron and inducing changes in muscle strength.[26] Dr. Omura had postulated that the changes in muscle strength are influenced by the light entering the eye and has noted that closing the eyes inhibits the test. The physiology of the O-ring requires further experiments with magnetic fields and the changes in intensity and frequency, and the activity of the pineal gland to further understand this process of resonance and finger strength. As in most things in science, this understanding may be updated with new information and experiments. Our authors have all agreed on this interpretation.

Dr. Omura conducted a series of experiments that support this resonance theory. Briefly, in the first experiment, he showed that two identical resonance circuits produced the same O-ring effect as two pure test substances (see Experiment I). In the second experiment, he placed a uni-directional diode between the patient's pointing finger and the test circuits and showed directionality (i.e., whether the "weakening" signal originates from the test substance or from the patient) (see Experiment II). In the third experiment, he introduced a laser beam into the basic setup to study the effects of a known test substance on a known carrier frequency and also showed forward and backward directionality (see Experiment III). In the fourth experiment, Omura investigated whether or not a test substance would transmit information in its electro-magnetic field (see Experiment IV).

EXPERIMENT I

In 1986, Dr. Omura suggested that the O-ring phenomenon must involve a resonance phenomenon between two separate electro-magnetic wave sources. [25 (p.127, 129, 130)] To test this hypothesis, instead of using two similar molecules he substituted two identical electro-magnetic resonance circuits with a constant inductance of one *microhenry* and a maximum variable capacitance of 75 Pico farads in series with no power source. A distance variable from a few centimeters to 200 meters separated these two circuits. He set the electro-magnetic resonance circuits to resonate at the same frequency and placed them perpendicular to each other, and they elicited a maximal opening of the O-ring. Electro-magnetic waves are transverse waves of magnetic and electric fields perpendicular to each other. The resonance circuits yield O-ring results identical to using identical test substances or identical molecules, which also evoke a weakening of the O-ring

EXPERIMENT II

In order to study whether the signal producing the ORT weakening response was going from the resonance circuit or "test substance" to the body or vice versa (thus, its directionality), Omura placed a germanium diode, IN34 [a uni-directional electronic component], between the patient and the nearest of the two electro-magnetic resonance circuits. There was no weakening response when the diode was "oriented in the forward direction from the fingertip to the resonance circuit." Conversely, there was a weakening response when that same diode was oriented in the opposite direction. Hence, this indicates that the signal detected by the O-ring test travels from the test substance to the body, and not vice versa.

EXPERIMENT III

Dr. Omura investigated whether the electro-magnetic field information of a test substance that was located within the patient's visual field, particularly in the area gazed upon, was transmitted to the patient's eyes. [25(pp130, 141)] A microscopic slide of pure alpha-streptococcus was placed in front of the patient at a predetermined distance.

a). When a strep-infected patient gazed at the microscopic slide, the O-ring test showed a weakened response, since the electro-magnetic field of the test substance is carried bi-directionally, consistent with Experiment III. Conversely, when all other conditions were kept the same but a book or metal sheet was placed in front of the patient, in order to obstruct the patient's view of the slide, the O-ring test did not show a weakened response.

b). When a non-strep-infected patient held a microscopic slide with alpha-strep in his hand while gazing at an identical microscopic slide at the same distance as above, the same O-ring test weakening response was observed.

Omura studied methodically (1) a waveform phenomenon, as was seen in the laser beam experiment, and (2) an electrical induction/conductance phenomenon, as seen with the electro-magnetic resonance circuits or metal wire conductors. Both techniques showed the carrying capability of both uni- and bi-directional electro-magnetic information, the form of information, and the perpendicular direction of transverse waves of electric and magnetic fields, which were consistent with electro-magnetism.

Another aspect concerning the basic mechanism of the O-ring method is that this phenomenon must involve the electro-magnetic resonance between separate electro-magnetic wave sources located inside and outside the body, or between a certain test substance held in the hand and an identical substance *in vivo* or *in vitro*. If the test substance and the substance to be examined have an identical molecular structure with the same stereo specificity, then both substances will emit electro-magnetic radiation of the same frequency and together can create a resonance phenomenon. [25 (p128)]

In summary, Omura had suggested, along with Takeshige, that the ability of humans to discriminate between two pure molecular substances through the O-ring derives from the electrical potential generated from the resonance. Then they discussed the signal's ability to travel through the central nervous system, including the *Nucleus Reticularis Giganto Cellularis* of the reticular formation, which gives negative feedback to the alpha-motor neurons in order for the O-ring test to produce a weakening response. [26(p131)] Similarly, an analogous human capability is demonstrated in the immunological response, which discriminates between self and non-self microorganisms and creates an immune response to the particular microorganism based upon its molecular structure. [27, 28] The bi-digital O-ring test discriminates between normal and abnormal tissue on the body and in it, and between substances of similar waveforms situated both outside and inside the body.

The experiments Omura conducted support the notion that the O-ring implicates phenomena similar to electro-magnetism and resonance and can be accurately reproduced with the scientific method. Without such an understanding, astonishing capabilities may be wrongly attributed to the examiner. These capabilities are innate and universally human, and it is through a scientific approach that they can be understood and used for diagnosis and treatment. It could be expressed as "bringing a diamond to the surface." However, individuals will be able to discriminate between things that have importance to them and that will prove very useful to people who want to understand something — dosages of a drug, vitamin or food — that may otherwise require great expense.

CHAPTER THREE
MATERIALS AND METHODS

BASIC O-RING TEST METHOD

The patient forms an O-ring shape by placing the tip of the thumb against the tip of the index finger of the same hand. The examiner attempts to open the patient's O-ring, as follows: With both forearms in front of his own chest and positioned in a straight horizontal line along the frontal plane, the examiner forms O-rings with the thumb and index fingers of each hand interlocking with the patient's O-ring.

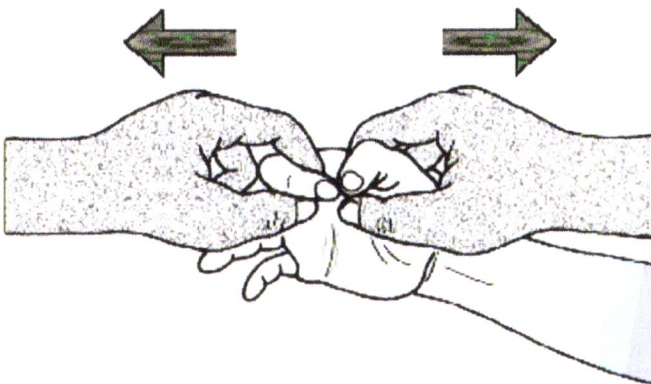

Figure 5A
Examiner's View

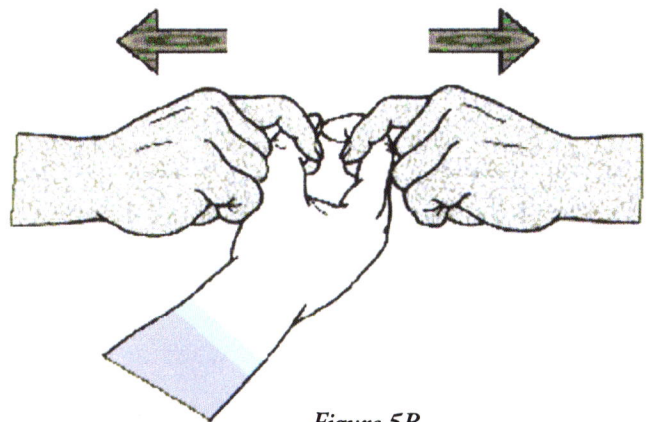

Figure 5B
Patient's View

The examiner then applies a moderate pulling motion in opposite directions along a straight line as indicated by the arrows shown in Figure 5B. The speed at which the examiner tries to pull the patient's two fingers apart is important. It should be a slow steady pull, not a fast jerking motion. The actual length of time during which the examiner pulls should not exceed three seconds; there should be a pause of at least six seconds before performing the next O-ring test. One should avoid a steady stream of pulls as this will yield false results because of a residual, or phantom, effect of the previous pull. [5(p61)]

DIRECT AND INDIRECT O-RING TESTING

There are two variations for applying the bi-digital O-ring test: direct and indirect. Direct testing involves the examiner and the patient (see Figure 2A, 2B). Indirect testing includes a third person as an intermediary, who is placed between the examiner and the patient (see Figure 3). This method is used when a patient is unwilling or unable to cooperate, e.g., as with an infant, an unconscious person, or an animal. For either variation, the basic O-ring method is used.

For the direct method, a non-conducting probe such as a wood or plastic rod, is used; for the indirect method, a conducting probe like a wire or a metal rod with a blunted tip that has a diameter of 1.0mm or less, should be used. For both methods, the probe should be placed perpendicular to the patient's skin at the location to be tested. Whether to use the direct or indirect method depends upon the reliability of the subject being used for the test. If a reliable third person is available to participate then the indirect method is the best approach. Obviously, testing an animal or incapacitated person requires the indirect method.

GENERAL CONSIDERATIONS TO INCREASE RELIABILITY

The examiner, the patient, and the third person must remove any metallic necklace, bracelet or watchband during the O-ring test procedures. The test may be done with the patient sitting or standing, and with the patient's neck maintained erect. When performing the test, the patient must keep his elbows at least 15 centimeters (6 inches) [5(p62)] away from his body so that the electromagnetic field of the kidneys does not bias the results. In other words just as one does not perform the ORT near an electrical or magnetic field such as an electric motor, the field of the kidneys can also bias the test results.

Prior to beginning, the examiner must determine whether there is any problem with the patient's neck. This is achieved by repeating the O-ring test using the most sensitive finger combination (see instructions in Table 1 and 2 below), with the patient's head in each of the following four positions:

The head bent forward
The head extended backward
The head rotated to the left
The head rotated to the right

If there is no change in the strength of the O-ring with the patient's head in each of the four positions the testing may begin. If the patient's O-ring weakens in any of the aforementioned positions the test will be unreliable unless the patient's head is maintained in a "straight ahead" position at all times with the eyes open. Maintaining a correct neck position is always a good idea when testing a subject because of possible cervical instability upon movement. Also, it is recommended that the subject looks at the same image throughout the testing.

PREPARATION FOR O-RING TESTING OF SUBSTANCES

Before proceeding with O-ring testing of substances, the examiner must determine which of the patient's thumb and finger combinations will produce the most accurate O-ring results. This finger combination is called the "most sensitive O-ring finger."

Some finger combinations will be too difficult to open; others will offer little resistance and are too weak. Therefore, the examiner should check the patient's O-ring finger combinations in succession:

Thumb with the index finger
Thumb with the middle finger
Thumb with the ring finger
Thumb with the little finger

The objective is to find the patient's or the third person's O-ring combination that will not open when the examiner pulls with his own O-rings formed by the thumb and index fingers of each hand, but will open when the examiner pulls with his own O-rings formed with thumb and index plus middle finger (three fingers) of each hand.

After determining the appropriate finger combination, for clinical convenience, a visual analogue scale (VAS) between –4 and +4 inclusive, is used to enable relative comparison of a test substance's influence. (See Table 1, 2) Once the "most sensitive O-ring finger" has been established a VAS may be assigned to the test results according to the relative width of the O-ring opening. (See Table 1)

The examiner may elect to use an alternate method of combining his "pulling" thumbs and fingers of both hands for determining the VAS results from –4 to –1(weakening response). (See Table 2)

The indirect method employs a third person so then all of the aforementioned steps to select the third person's most sensitive finger combination must be performed. The third person must use a metal probe — preferably aluminum or copper, to lightly touch the patient's skin surface perpendicularly at the location to be tested. Omura demonstrated that there is a weakening of the patient's O-ring while holding a control substance under the following conditions — while the patient is:

Pointing a finger toward a similar substance at short distances of less than one-third meter.
Staring at a similar substance that is placed nearby. [25(pp130,139,141)]
Holding and placing a copper wire near or on a similar substance.

According to Omura, the fingers and eyes both can detect an intensified electro-magnetic field, which carries information within the emitted field (see below). [25(p139,141)]

PROCEDURE FOR TESTING SUBSTANCES

When all the conditions mentioned above are satisfied, the examiner may begin the formal procedure for testing various substances.

The patient, or the third person, holds the test substance in his/her free hand. (A test substance can be *in vitro* or *in vivo*; for example, a microscopic slide of human organ tissue, bacteria, virus, monoclonal antibodies, neurotransmitter, cancer tissue, toxin, fungus, parasites, etc., or an organ representation point on the surface of the body, i.e. Mu or Shu point.) Areas of the patient's skin are stimulated by lightly touching them with a probe, held perpendicularly to the patient's skin by the patient or a third person. During the direct method the skin of the patient could be stimulated by a piece of band-aid, a small suction cup, etc, if the area that needs stimulation is difficult to reach by the patient's free hand (i.e. the back).

The patient's O-ring will open if a "resonance" exists between the test substance and the area of skin on the patient that is stimulated, i.e., lightly touched, by the probe. With both the direct and indirect methods, this indicates that a similar substance is present in the area of the patient's body being contacted by the probe.

Additionally, while holding the control substance in the hand, it can be compared to another substance that is outside the body by using a wire or pointing a finger at the outside substance.

VAS BI-DIGITAL O-RING RESPONSE.

TABLE 1		TABLE 2	
Criteria for assignment of numerical VAS according to bi-digital O-ring test responses		Alternate criteria for assignment of numerical VAS according to bi-digital O-ring test responses	
	VAS Bi-digital O-Ring Response		VAS Bi-digital O-Ring Response
-4	O-ring opens completely when the examiner uses only one finger * of each hand (= maximal weakening response)	-4	O-ring opens completely when the examiner uses one finger of each hand (= maximal weakening response)
-3	Opens three-quarters when the examiner uses only one finger	-3	Opens completely when the examiner uses 2 fingers
-2	Opens one-half when the examiner uses only one finger	-2	Opens completely when the examiner uses 3 fingers
-1	Opens one-quarter when the examiner uses only one finger	-1	Opens completely when the examiner uses 4 fingers
+1	O-ring remains closed when the examiner uses one finger of each hand		Note: the following criteria are identical to Table 1
		+1	O-ring remains closed when the examiner uses one finger of each hand
+2	Remains closed when the examiner uses 2 fingers	+2	Remains closed when the examiner uses 2 fingers
+3	Remains closed when the examiner uses 3 fingers	+3	Remains closed when the examiner uses 3 fingers
+4	Remains closed, even when the examiner uses 4 fingers*	+4	Remains closed, even when the examiner uses 4 fingers*

* Finger(s): This designation refers to use of fingers(s) plus the thumb forming the O-ring. The thumb does not count as a finger. [7]

NEW GAUGING SYSTEM FOR THE CANCER SCREENING

In the last few years Dr. Omura has adopted a new gauging system in the procedure of cancer and Alzheimer screening. The new cancer screening method is performed with the help of a third person holding a reference cancer marker (Integrin-α1 or β-Amyloid in case of Alzheimer) in the proximity of a laser beam. The beam is directed at a series of body points from a distance of 15 to 20 feet and the data are recorded. The gauging is a bit different than the classic one already described. The operator starts with his/her O-rings formed by the thumb and the index finger and the O-ring formed by the thumb and the ring finger of the third person.

This first position would be +1 if it opens.
Next the O-ring formed by the thumb and the middle finger of the third person. This would be +2 if it opens.
Next the O-Ring formed by the thumb and the index finger of the third person. This would be +3 if it opens.

Now the third person would keep forming the O-ring with their thumb and index finger while the operator would use the O-rings formed by the thumb and the middle finger:
This would be +4 if it opens.
Next the O-rings formed by the thumb and the ring finger of the operator. This would be +5 if it opens.
Last the O-rings formed by the thumb and the fifth finger of the operator. This would be +6 if it opens.

The result would be interpreted this way:
+1 & +2 negative
+3 & +4 moderate positive or suspect
+5 & +6 positive 34

This would be +1 if it opens.
Next the O-Ring formed by the thumb and the middle finger. This would be +2 if it opens.
Next the O-Ring formed by the thumb and the index finger. This would be +3 if it opens.

Now the third person would keep forming the O-ring with the thumb and the index finger and the operator would use the O-rings formed by the thumb and the middle finger:

This would be +4 if it opens
Next the O-rings formed by the thumb and the ring finger. This would be +5 if it opens.
Last the O-rings formed by the thumb and the fifth finger. This would be +6 if it opens.

The result would be interpreted this way:
+1 & +2 negative
+3 & +4 moderate positive or suspect
+5 & +6 positive

CHAPTER FOUR
IMPORTANT DISCOVERIES
PART I: TRADITIONAL CHINESE MEDICINE

This chapter elucidates part of Dr. Omura's contribution to Traditional Chinese Medicine, TCM, 中医, zhongyi. Some of the mappings of the *umunculus* and pathways he found in various parts of the body will be presented. Some examples are multiple pathways of the stomach meridian, a deviation from the starting point in the heart; and pathways from all internal organs passing through areas of the cranium.

In the 1980s Shinnick decided to do an independent analysis of the meridian pathway of TCM without Omura's help, knowledge or guidance. Some of these experiments will be presented here. Clinical testing with patients will be illustrated in Chapter 6.

The previous chapter summarizes the discovery, development, technique, and theory of Omura's Bi-digital O-ring phenomenon, which provides a sensitive diagnostic screening method now applied widely in Western and Oriental medicine. Omura theorized this as an electro-magnetic phenomenon and provided experiments to support it. The O-ring can also be used to identify internal and external pathology and to locate traditional meridian pathways and boundaries of internal organs.

The following pictures are the organ representation points of the back (SHU) and front (MU) (Figure 6), the stomach meridian (figure 7), the thymus network of women (figure 8), the umunculus of the tongue (figure 9), and the hand (figure 10A and 10B) imaged by Omura and compiled by Borgna and Shinnick from workshops and clinical cases.

In 1984 Omura demonstrated that by touching a subject's organ representation point, like the stomach, [Ren 12 (Front-Mu or Alarm point zhongwan中腕)] with a non-conducting probe while the subject was simultaneously holding a substance like aspirin — known to be toxic to that organ — the O-ring test produces a weakening response. This confirmed the relationship between the Mu points and their respective organs as described in Traditional Chinese Medicine. (Figure 6)

In 1985 Omura showed that with the subject holding a microscopic slide of a specific organ tissue as a *reference control substance*, a meridian-like pathway of that internal organ could be mapped or "imaged" on the surface of the skin.

In the beginning experiments used aspirin as the control substance, which showed an opening of the O-ring. As a known toxin this proved that the organs responded to a control substance, or body location and one could detect and map pathways.

The stomach meridian 胃经 weijing starts in the face, just below the center of the eye, and has multiple pathways going out from the stomach and across the abdomen. While only one pathway can be seen in the traditional charts, the O-Ring method showed multiple channels diverging and converging to the main pathway. See Figure 7.

In 1987, Omura's publications demonstrated that six of 12 traditional meridians could be detected not only by a reference control substance of its related organ (e.g. microscopic slide of stomach tissue for the stomach meridian), but also by the control substance of the preceding organ or pair organ. That is, the first of two organs that comprise a yin-yang "organ/pair system" (e.g. with the microscopic spleen slide you can detect the spleen and the stomach meridian). For example, lung precedes large intestine, spleen precedes stomach, heart precedes small intestine, etc. "The reverse does not work; with the microscopic stomach slide, the spleen meridian cannot be imaged, and so on." [22(p56)]

Figure 6A, Mu (Alarm) Points

Mu Points
1   TMJ
2   Thyroid
3   Thymus
4   Lungs
5   Heart
6   Diaphragm
7   Liver
8   Gallbladder
9   Stomach
10   Pancreas
11   Ascending colon
12   Small intestine
13   Descending colon
14   Ureter
15   Urinary bladder
16a Ovary
16b Testes
17   Uterus
18   Prostate
19   Kidney
20   Neck vascular points
21   Lung points
22   Cardiovascular points (bladder points identified)

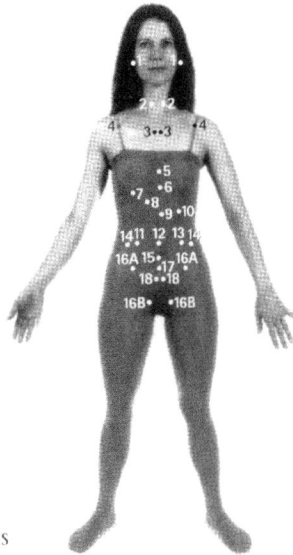

Figure 6B, Shu Points

Shu Points

Vertebra	Organ
5	Liver
6	Spleen
7	Gallbladder
8	Stomach
8 (lower)	Duodenum
9	Pancreas
10	Adrenal gland
11	Colon

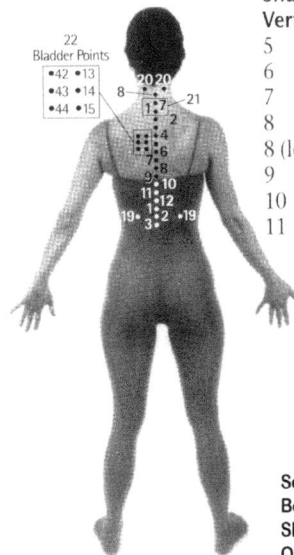

Source: 1992 Adriano Borgna, M.D., and Phillip Shinnick, Ph.D. from Omura Seminars.

Figure 6
Organ Representation Points on the front (mu) and back (shu) [16(p.245)]

Along with these relationships Omura found that the pericardium meridian could be detected with the adrenal gland tissue sample and the triple warmer meridian by the ovaries and testes tissue samples. He also found that the SA node tissue sample can be used to detect the AV node.

According to Omura, the starting point of the heart (1), Jiquan, is not in the axilla but further up on the arm.

Omura used thymus tissue samples to detect its network. The internal network has long been charted by western science but not the external one. Later Omura re-evaluated his network and found a much more elaborate network on the mammary glands' thymus support system. [23, 31] See Figure 8.

In testing the *umunculus* in various parts of the body Omura experimented with the use of hormone samples produced by various organs as reference substances and found a correspondence with the weakening of the O-Ring, which represents a resonance between two substances. Examples are: *natriuretic peptide* could identify heart areas; *gastrin* the stomach; *ovaries* and *testosterone estrone, estriol, progesterone*; etc….correspond to the triple warmer organ system of TCM. [29, 30]

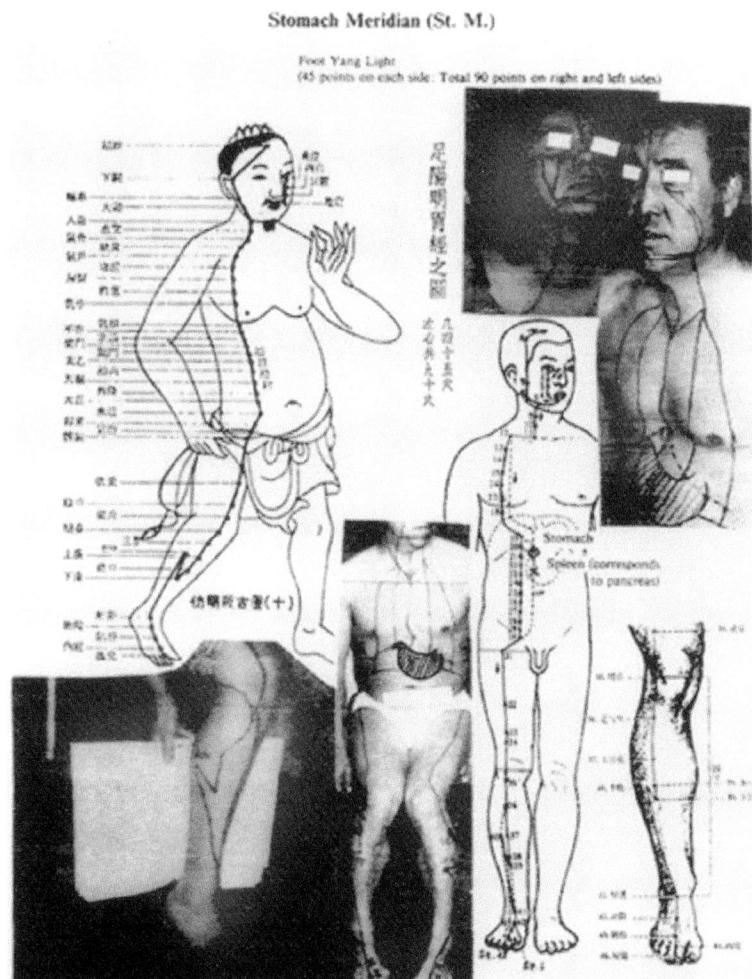

Figure 7 Stomach Meridian showing multiple pathways from the stomach [30, 36(p. 165), 22(p.59)]
This figure is reproduced with special permission of Yoshiaki Omura, M.D.,Sc.D.

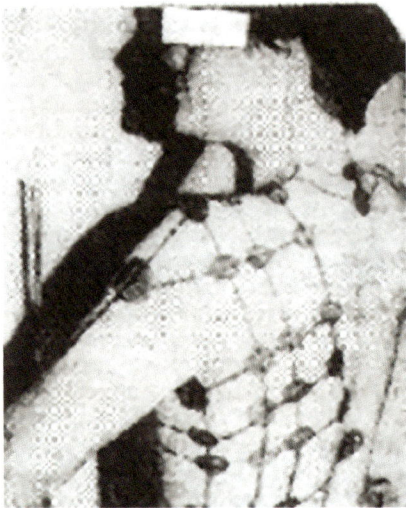

Figure 8, Case A [31A(p. 81, 7C)]
Back view
Thymus

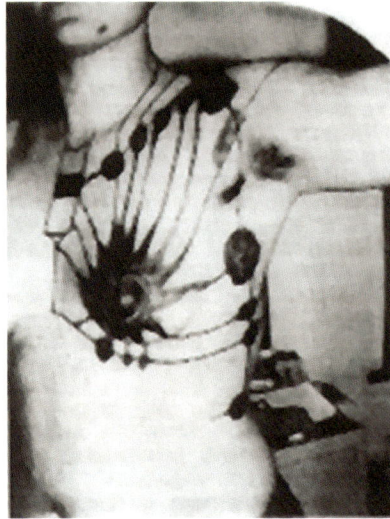

Figure 8, Case A [31A(p. 81, 7B)]
Front view
Thymus

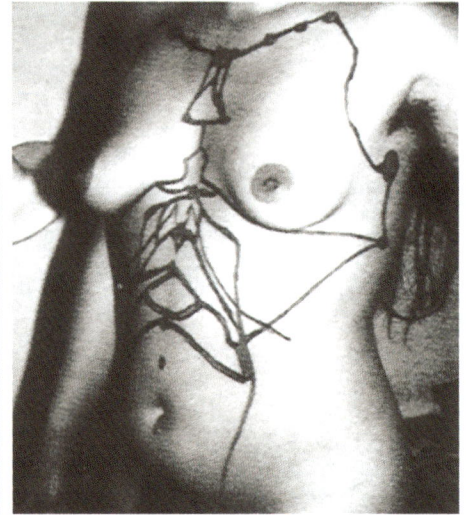

Figure 8a, Case B [23, 31(p. 5), 31A(p. 81, 7A)]
Front view
Thymus

These figure are reproduced with special permission of Yoshiaki Omura, M.D.,Sc.D.

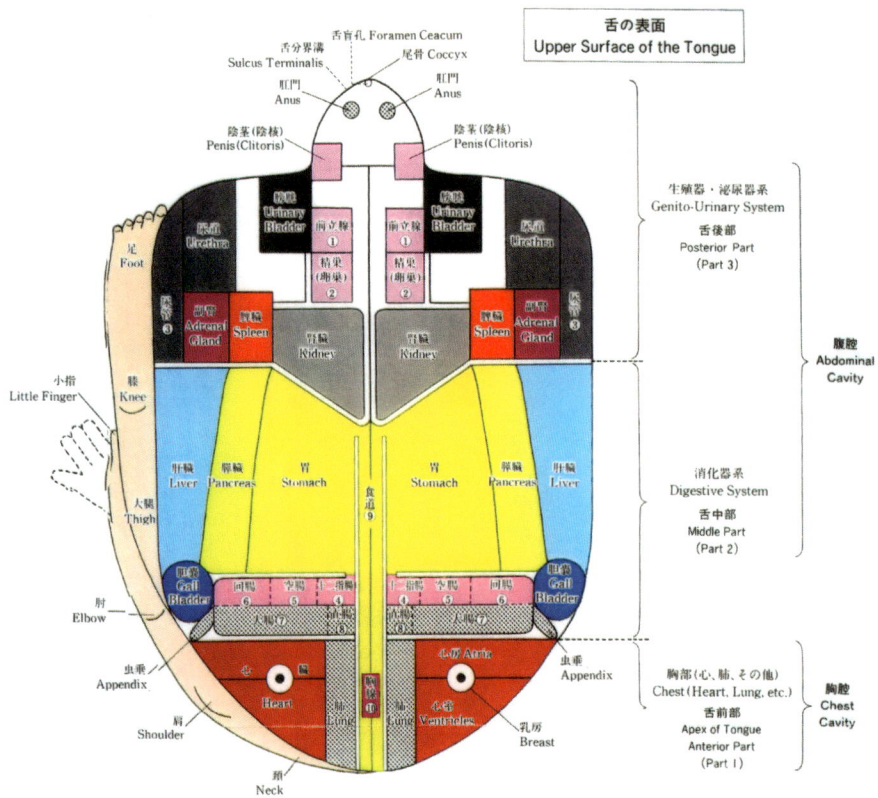

Figure 9 Tongue [32(p. 34)]
This figure is reproduced with special permission of Yoshiaki Omura, M.D.,Sc.D.

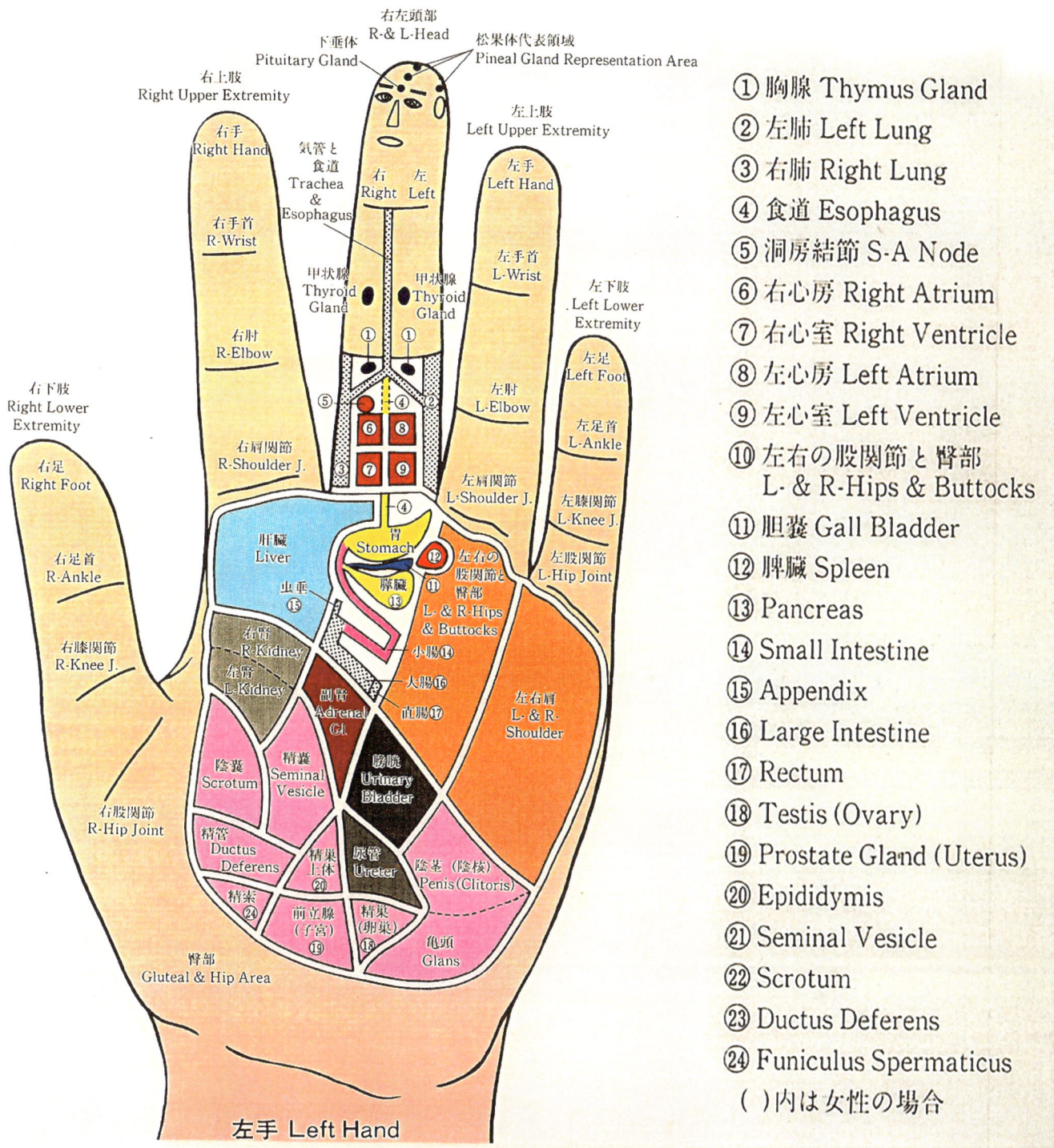

Figure 10A Omura Imaging of Left Hand [33]
This figure is reproduced with special permission of Yoshiaki Omura, M.D.,Sc.D.

① 胸腺 Thymus Gland
② 左肺 Left Lung
③ 右肺 Right Lung
④ 食道 Esophagus
⑤ 洞房結節 S-A Node
⑥ 右心房 Right Atrium
⑦ 右心室 Right Ventricle
⑧ 左心房 Left Atrium
⑨ 左心室 Left Ventricle
⑩ 左右の股関節と臀部 L- & R-Hips & Buttocks
⑪ 胆嚢 Gall Bladder
⑫ 脾臓 Spleen
⑬ Pancreas
⑭ Small Intestine
⑮ Appendix
⑯ Large Intestine
⑰ Rectum
⑱ Testis (Ovary)
⑲ Prostate Gland (Uterus)
⑳ Epididymis
㉑ Seminal Vesicle
㉒ Scrotum
㉓ Ductus Deferens
㉔ Funiculus Spermaticus
（ ）内は女性の場合

21

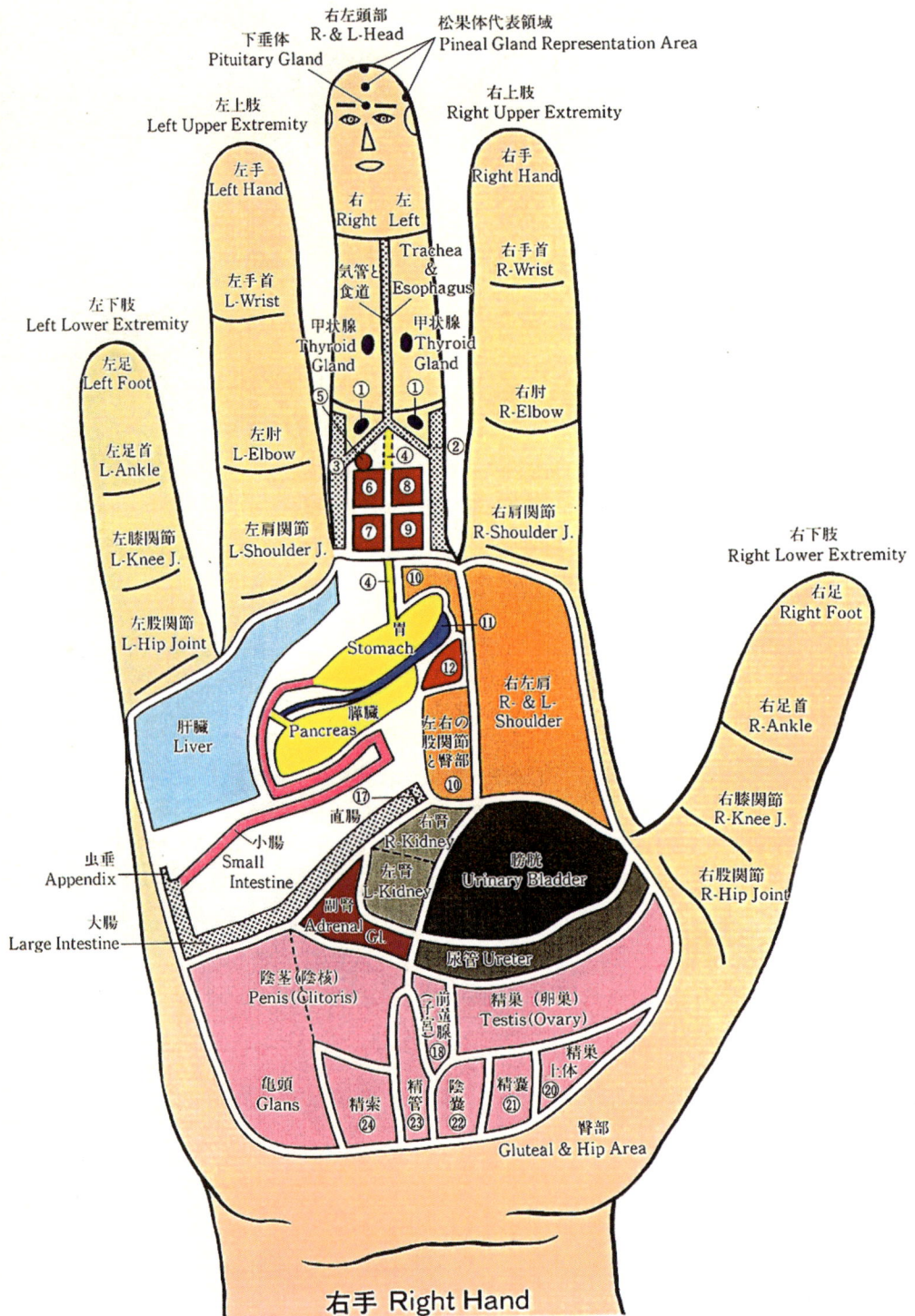

Figure 10B Omura Imaging of Right Hand [33]
This figure is reproduced with special permission of Yoshiaki Omura, M.D.,Sc.D.

22

CHAPTER FIVE
SHINNICK'S INDEPENDENT ASSESSMENT

I wanted to make an independent assessment of the O-ring and see if a disease or abnormal organ could be imaged, like Omura did with the normal organ tissue. The consensus of those familiar with Omura's work was that it had to be tested.

IMAGING OF TOXIC ORGAN PATHWAYS

In 1986, with the assistance of Celia Blumenthal, M.D. and Herbert Berger, Dipl OBT, I did this for the lung, with a cigar as the toxic substance taped to the wrist and the Mu Lung point as the control reference. This triple blind technique resulted in an imaged lung pathway lateral to the normal traditional lung pathway, with spheres along the pathway. The 1986 results are shown in Figure 11a and 11b. Our experiments had to be done on a pathway not previously imaged by Omura and the technique had to be blind, i.e. the subject, experimenter and assistant could not see what each was doing.

The toxic lung below was imaged in 1986, the normal lung in 1991, and the normal colon in 1987. [4] (Figure 12) The colon can be imaged by using either lung or colon tissue. The toxic colon was only imaged up to the shoulder. We also compared the normal and toxic lungs. (Figure 12A,B,C) These are superimposed upon each other and shown below.

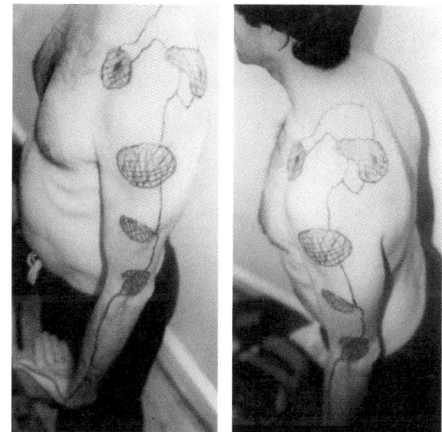

Figure 11A and 11B 1986
Triple blind study with Lung Mu Point
肺*(Zhongfu) and Cigar as a Toxin*
The microscopic slides of organ tissues were obtained from Carolina Biological Supply Co., Burlington, NC

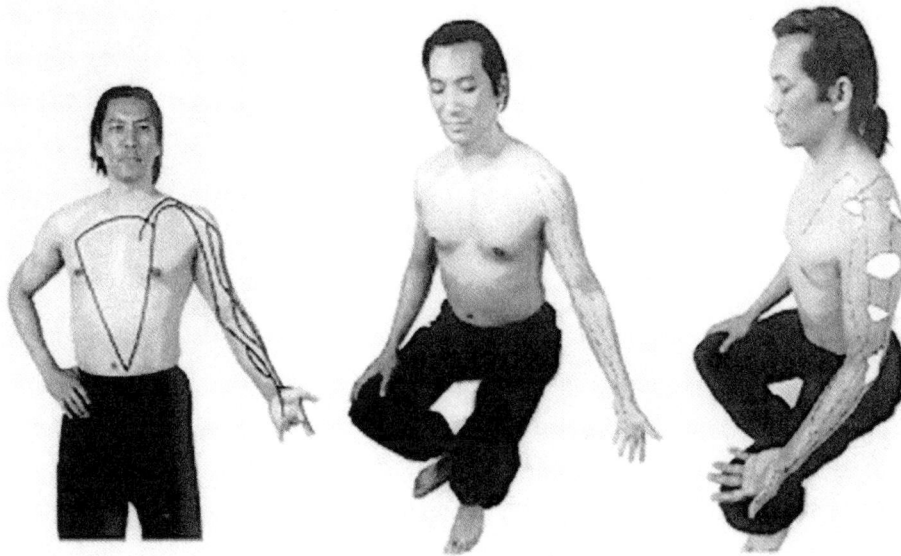

Figure 12

12A Lung (lateral) and Colon (medial)
12B Toxic Colon Figure
12C Lung (medial) and Toxic Lung (lateral)

There is a junction on the forearm of the lung pathway that deviates toward a lateral pathway when a known lung toxin is added. Could this deviation occur if there is a blockage on the surface of the pathway? To test this a germanium diode, which only flows in one direction, was put above the junction. Figure 13 reflects that experiment. The blocked flow deviated to the toxic pathway. A germanium diode NTE 109 from NTE Electronics, Bloomfield, New Jersey (PRV-100 Max Vf-10V @ 200mA IF-2oomA) was used to determine direction by simply placing it on the pathway. If placed in the wrong direction then the pathway could not be imaged beyond the diode. However, in the right direction the pathway appeared as usual.

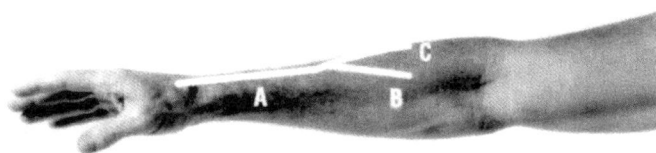

Figure 13

Lung Pathway Blocked by a Diode.
Normal pathway from A to B, blocked, goes to C.

What would happen if there was a scar along the organ pathway or the organ itself was impaired? Figure's 14A and 14B reflect this. A patient with a recent mastectomy complained of constant constipation. The colon pathway was imaged in Figure 14A with the original pathway superimposed on a model. Her constipation was relieved immediately after acupuncture to the pathway and maintained for months. Then she had a breast replacement (Figure 14B.) The nipple from the good breast was excised, cut into two pieces, and put on the nipple-less scarred breast. A saline implant was inserted to give the breast mass. Her constipation came back, probably due to the disturbances of the colon pathway located on the anterior thoracic chest from chemotherapy. (See next chapter for chemotherapy effects on organs.) The colon pathway 结肠经 jiechang jing was imaged and acupunctured along the pathway, then re-imaged as shown below in Figures 14B and 14C. Also, she received acupuncture on the Shu Point in the back at the 11th thoracic vertebrae. This produced a more permanent relief of her constipation. Another treatment was given five months later, presented in Figure 14D, showing a lateral shift to a more normal pathway. Then four months later, as shown in Figure 14E, a partial imaging shows a shift to the right for constipation after acupuncture, further toward the nipple. After that she received acupuncture for constipation about once a year for three years. Two other cases presented with constipation and reported silicone breast implants; they imaged similar to Figure 14E. See Chapter Six, for details of this case study testing cancer substance treatment.

CHANGES IN PATHWAYS DUE TO SURGICAL INTERVENTION

Colon Imaging of Cancer Patient with Breast Reconstruction 1987-1988

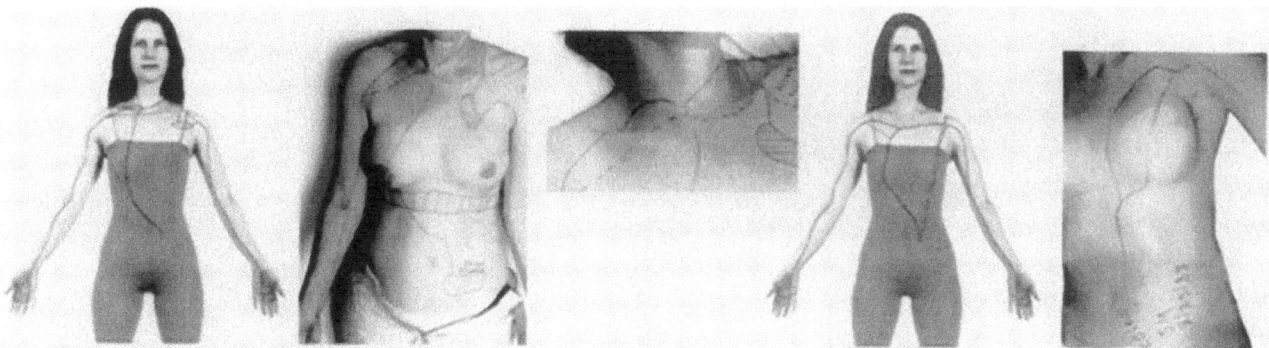

Figure 14A	*Figure 14B*	*Figure 14C*	*Figure 14D*	*Figure 14E*
Mastectomy	*Breast reconstruction*	*After Acupuncture*	*After Acupuncture*	*After Acupuncture*
Colon Imaging	*Colon Imaging*	*11/87*	*4/1/88*	*8/25/88*
8/87 Model	*11/87 Patient*	*Dotted line Colon Imaging*		*Shifted to right*
				Colon Imaging

What would happen to the lung pathway if the organ were impaired or had some pathology? Figure 15 reflects a patient who had 60% of his left lung removed because of alder poisoning from a wood workshop-processing job. The lung pathway imaged very similar to the toxic pathway and the differences can be explained by the technique used to image the pathway. Originally, to image the pathways the organ representation point (ORP), or Mu point for the lung (see Figure 11) was stimulated. In this patient lung tissue was used and the difference in technique resulted in a pathway that goes toward the cervical more than the organ representation point (ORP), as in Figure 15. (See Figure 17B, which shows a difference between the modern lung pathway that goes to the lung Mu point — as in our Figure 11— and a pathway from the Ming dynasty that is more like the pathway imaged with tissue). Both techniques are useful; using the ORP means you do not have to use lung tissue, when a sample of lung tissue is not available. Below, in Figure 15 using ogran tissue, the pathway is shown before and after electrical stimulation with surface electrodes.

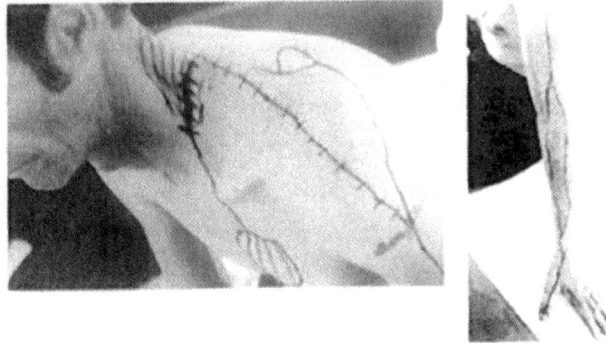

Figure 15A, 15B
Figure 15A 1987 Lung.
After electrical stimulation cross marked line
Figure 15B 1987 Lung

Electrical parameter: WQ10B stimulator. Made in the People's Republic of China. (The negative parameters are listed in parenthesis) Rise Time 15 μsec (5 μsec), Fall Time 5 μsec (5 μsec), Z out = 2k (40), Max 120V (-15V -12.5 V), 40 μsec at 63% Amp. (420 μsec) (8).

Another toxic lung pathway was found in 1989 when a patient complained of tingling sensations in her shoulders, neck stiffness of Cervical Vertebra-2 (C-2), depression, and numbness in her fingers. Motor fiber conduction tests showed C-7, Thoracic Vertebra-1 (T-1) muscle membrane instability. A MRI showed no abnormality. She was being exposed to Besting, a photograph-processing toxin, and had two auto accidents. The diagnosis was ulnar neuropathy and fibromyalgia. Testing of the lung Mu point 肺 fei showed abnormality and, suspecting a lung toxin, we imaged her lung pathway from the Mu point (ORP) rather than using a microscopic slide of lung tissue.

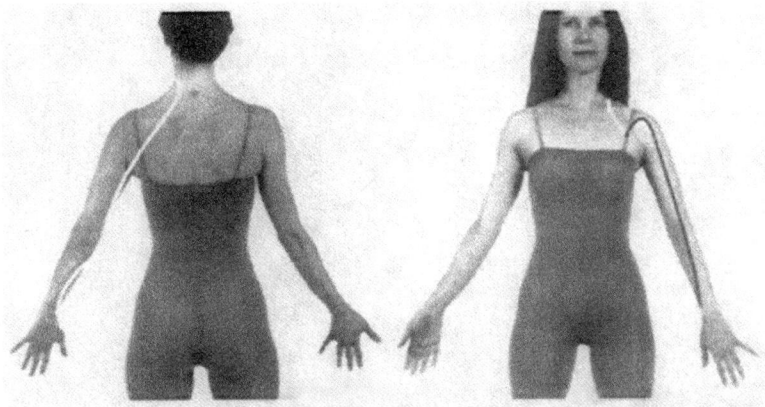

Before acupuncture   *After acupuncture*
16A 1989 Lung from Mu point (white line)
16B 1989 Lung from Mu point after acupuncture. (black line)

This leaves open many questions as to the location of lung and colon, which seem to be reversed according to the Modern Traditional Chinese Main Meridian System 中医主经络系统 zhongyi zhu jingluo xitong, which is shown below. However, further comparing the pathways to the Ming Dynasty Meridian from the shoulder, there is compatibility below the elbow, although this may vary according to the individual. Also below the elbow a rotation is a possibility, the position is not fixed, and the same could be said about the thumb. Natural variations in position result in energy or chi variation.

COMPARISON TO MODERN AND ANCIENT MERIDIAN CHARTS

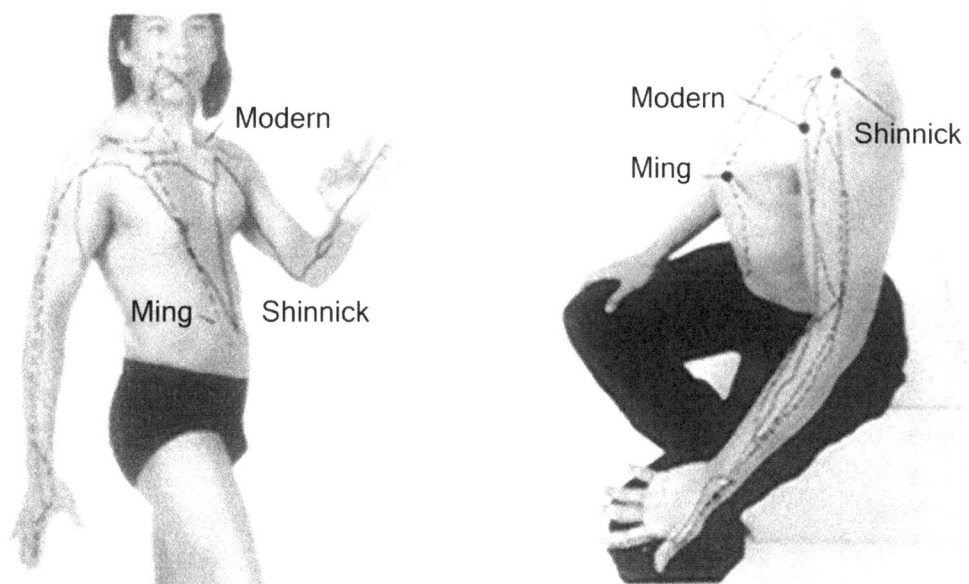

Figure 17

17A Shinnick Colon pathway compared to Modern and Ming Dynasty.
17B Shinnick Lung pathway compared to Modern and Ming dynasty

Figure 17A needs some explanation. Three electronically layered pathways are presented for the colon. The Modern pathway is a dotted line, the Ming pathway is a spaced line, and Shinnick's pathway is a continuous line.[7] The Shinnick and Ming pathways generally match across the chest, with the Modern and Ming going to the face. The Modern and Ming generally match on the arm. Below the shoulder, the Shinnick goes palmar. Figure 17B is a general match except for the starting position in the hand. The modern meridian system coincides with our imaging by means of the Mu point of the lung, while the more ancient meridian system coincides with our imaging with organ tissue as illustrated above.

The big difference is the colon pathway. The author's is more medial, where the modern and Ming pathways appear in the radial front of the arm. Since the Shinnick pathway was done blind and at random the difference may be individual, since there is a rotating forearm below the elbow. Also, as shown with the toxic lung pathway, an imaging of a random subject may show a sub-clinical colon abnormality in the imaging. It is interesting to note that the bifurcation of the lung pathway in the Shinnick image shadows the modern and the Ming, combined with variations.

CHAPTER SIX
IMPORTANT DISCOVERIES;
PART II MODERN MEDICINE

APPLICATIONS FOR ORT TO CARDIOVASCULAR SYNDROMES

Using a microscopic slide of a particular artery Omura was able to accurately trace areas of brain circulation through certain arteries (posterior, anterior and medial). With the subject wearing a latex cap (like the one for swimming) he was able to draw the contours of the arteries on it and show areas of abnormality. Often acupuncture along the restricted artery could reestablish a good circulation and relieve the symptoms. He developed a technique to measure the blood pressure of the supra-orbital artery on the forehead surface by a special inflatable head cuff with a Doppler flow-measurement–device that he invented. He demonstrated that one could have high blood pressure in the arm and low blood pressure in the brain or high pressure on one side of the brain and low pressure on the other side. Relief of symptoms came from acupuncture around the areas of one or both of the posterior vertebral arteries, located along the side of the cervical spine at the level of the 6th cervical vertebra or carotid arteries, which are often narrowed due to tense muscles in the neck or one side of the neck. He called this Cephalic Hypo-tension Syndrome that can cause headaches, sleep disturbance, memory loss, irritability and changes in pain threshold. He linked these syndromes to hypoglycemia (pancreas) or liver and kidney problems. This may explain why high-blood pressure medications can have conflicting results. Lowering the B/P may exacerbate some of the symptoms because the patient may have a local hypotension. These images by Omura are important for therapists dealing with patients' vascular circulation spasticity to recognize asymmetry in blood flow bifurcation due to hypertension.

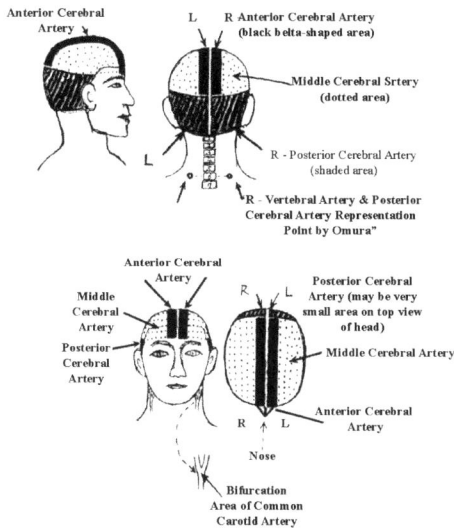

Figure 18A cerebral brain circulation
Mapping organs on the head with a latex cap [34(p. 146)]
Picture by Omura

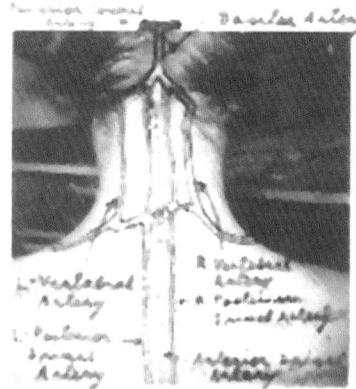

Figure 18B
Mapping of posterior cerebral
circulation [35(p. 156)]

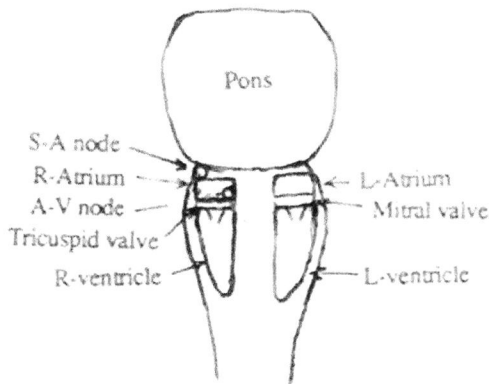

Heart representation areas in medulla
oblongata in individuals with normal
blood pressure

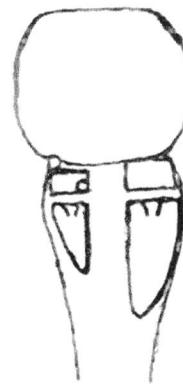

Heart representation areas in medulla
oblongata in hypertensive individuals

18C
Mapping of the heart representation areas on the back of the neck over the
medulla oblongata of separate individuals for changes in size according to normal and hypertension.
These figures are reproduced with special permission of Yoshiaki Omura, M.D.,Sc.D.

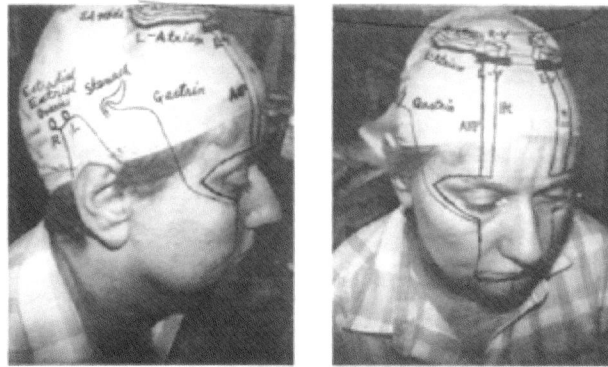

18D
Stomach and heart representation points on cranium [36(p. 164)]
This figure is reproduced with special permission of Yoshiaki Omura, M.D.,Sc.D.

Application of these principles led to taking blood pressure at the level of the supra-orbital artery to determine cephalic hypotension syndrome and asymmetry of the brain circulation. This was done with a special inflatable headband and Doppler flow meter developed by Omura. Shinnick, Freed, Blumenthal and Omura wrote about this, which is summarized below.

B/P is routinely measured at the level of the brachial artery. Omura was not satisfied with this method of measurement and devised his own. The first thing he did was to invent different sizes of cuffs that could be used at the level of the forehead and at the ankle. The second was to use a Doppler connected with an electronic amplifier instead of a stethoscope in order to make the measurement more objective. This new approach enabled him to have accurate B/P readings at different levels of the body (e.g. supra-orbital artery and tibial or pedial artery).

Figure 19 Omura drawing [2(p. 14)]

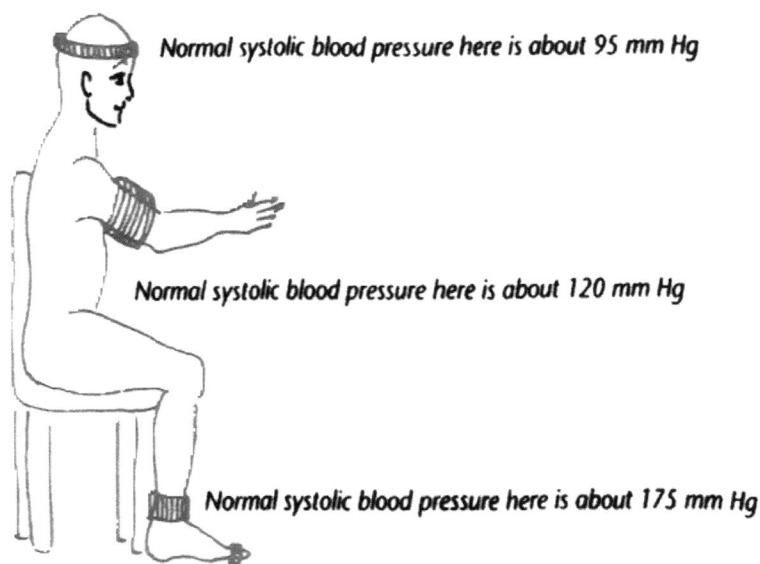

Normal systolic blood pressure here is about 95 mm Hg

Normal systolic blood pressure here is about 120 mm Hg

Normal systolic blood pressure here is about 175 mm Hg

Diagram 5   Blood pressure measurements at different points of the body.

This figure is reproduced with special permission of Yoshiaki Omura, M.D.,Sc.D.

As Omura explored blood pressure variations throughout the body, he reasoned that gravitational forces would cause differences in blood pressure readings. For example, blood flows down from the heart to the feet, and gravity acts to increase the pressure of the stream as it falls. By extensive experimentation and measurement, Omura verified that blood pressure in fact increases by 7.7 millimeters of mercury for each 10 centimeters of vertical distance from the heart level downward (toward the feet), and decreases by 7.7 millimeters for each 10 centimeters of vertical distance from the heart level upward (toward the head) in a subject in a standing or sitting position.

Although 120/80 is considered the "normal" blood pressure at the level of the brachial artery, there is no similar standard blood pressure in any other area of the body (120/80 is actually the normal blood pressure at the level of the heart). Taking this as a standard and using Omura's formula, one can calculate the "normal" expected blood pressure in any part of the body if the vertical distance from the heart is known. The actual pressure when measured using the Doppler may be higher, lower, or equivalent to this value. A deviation of more than 20% from the extrapolated value generally indicates pathology in an area.

In a normal individual who is lying down, the expected arterial blood pressure throughout the body would be uniform. However, for reasons unique to an individual, there may be differences between each side of the body even in the horizontal position. In experimenting with this new method Dr. Omura found that a normal B/P at the brachial artery does not mean normal B/P in other parts of the body. This observation has profound implications when it comes to the effect of medications that are commonly used in treating High B/P. If a patient is taking medication to lower his or her B/P it may exacerbate some of the problems (symptoms) due to a local hypotension (low B/P). Scientists at the Heart Disease Research Foundation believe that blood pressure should be routinely measured at multiple body sites in order to achieve a more effective diagnosis and treatment of circulatory problems.

In general, patients with asymmetric B/P readings, especially when the patterns were caused by asymmetrical posture, and asymmetry due to previous traumas or stress, quickly responded to acupuncture given to the area where the narrowing of the artery had been detected by BDORT. In several cases there was no response or a weak response to acupuncture, probably due to some undetectable internal factors related to other organ systems.

In several cases of older patients who developed arrhythmia due to emotional stress, acupuncture to the heart organ representation points as shown in the Mu and Shu Points, and to the thoracic rib cage quickly resolved arrhythmia. This phenomenon was confirmed in other patients as well. Almost invariably ORT will show asymmetry and spasticity in the neck area and resulting asymmetrical circulation disturbances when clinical symptoms like pain are present.

(18D) Omura, using various tissue samples, was able to map the umunculus on each side of the cranium and within the umunculus area of the heart as well as the SA and AV nodes, ventricle, and atria. He was also able to map it over the back of the neck where the area of medulla oblongata is located. In one patient he described the abnormalities in size of one side of the heart representation. (18C) He also described an umunculus on the lips, ears, feet, and tongue.

Once Omura realized that with the correspondent microscopic slide (e.g. microscopic slide of the stomach) it was possible to follow the entire meridian system of that particular organ he decided to verify the traditional meridian pathways shown in many traditional drawings. In most cases his findings were exactly the same as the traditional drawings, although the pathways he described were often more complex and with many more branches than the traditional ones, but there were a few exceptions.

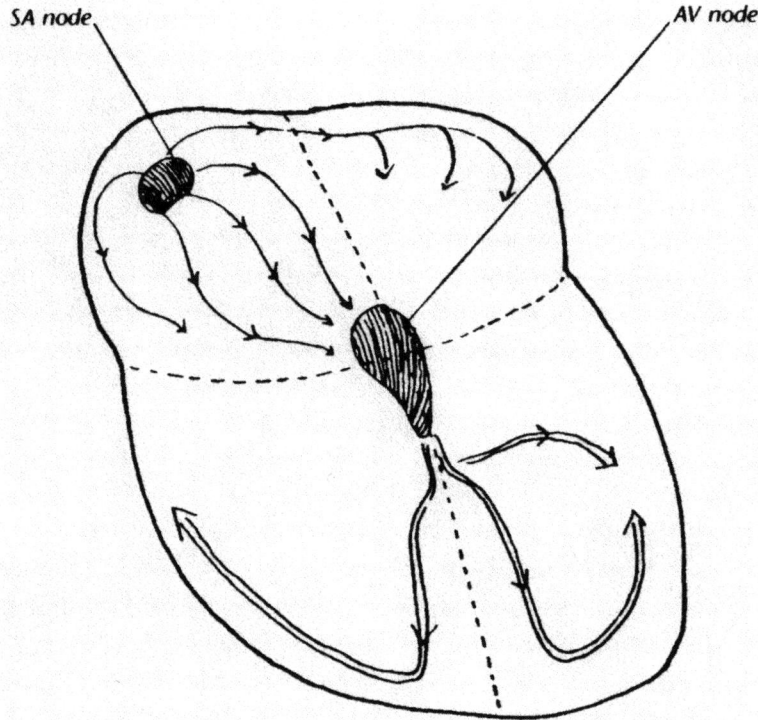

Diagram 6   *The sinoatrial (SA) node and the atrioventricular (AV) node are the two primary pacemaker cell groups in the heart. In a normal heart, the AV node follows the rhythm of the SA node. During a heart attack the spread of these electrical impulses (represented by the arrows in the diagram) is disrupted. The EKG, which reflects the spread of the electrical impulse, is useful in delineating areas of cardiac damage.*

Drawing by Celia Blumenthal, M.D.

Figure 20 [2(p. 17)]

FOOD AND DRUG COMPATIBILITY TO PATHOGENIC MICROORGANISMS

A practical application of the O-ring is in helping patients test the appropriate multi-vitamins or supplements. The procedure is simple. First the patient is tested for reliability by the normal procedure we described in Chapter 1 for the direct ORT; then simply the control substance (vitamin or supplement) is placed in the hand of the patient that is free. If the ring formed with the most sensitive finger opens, the substance is not helpful for that individual. If the same ring becomes stronger the substance it is helpful. The change in strength of the ring is also dosage related, so you may observe no change in strength with one dosage but you may notice a change if the dosage is increased or decreased.

A 1986 CASE STUDY

DETAILED ANALYSIS OF A BREAST CANCER PATIENT

In 1986 (Figure 14) Dr. Omura, assisted by Dr. Shinnick, examined a patient who had been diagnosed with breast cancer and had a radical mastectomy. Post operational radiological diagnostic procedures showed shadows on her left upper quadrant in an area operated on indicating a possible spread of the cancer. She was undergoing chemotherapy. The O-ring evaluation showed abnormalities in blood flow to the brain due to the position of the neck in the head up, down and turning to the left position. Fluctuations of the blood flow in these cervical positions were also correlated with O-Ring abnormalities of the thymus and thyroid. In other words her cervical problems caused the thymus and thyroid to function or not function according with the position of the neck. The medial cerebral artery area showed a –4 as well as the anterior cerebral artery on the left side. Spasticity of the muscle around the cervical vertebrae 6-7 on the left side and trapezius and abnormality of the thyroid gland were also noticed.

Cancer test showed anti- Necrosis Tumor Factor NTF CEA (Carcinoembryonic Antigen)-EIA method O-Ring Test for infections found:
- *Clamydia*–4 to the head, neck, throat, vagina, breast.
- *Syphilis* to nose, mouth and throat.
- *Neisseria gonorrhea* to the throat, bladder, thoracic duct, posterior left brain, occipital.

The antibiotic, *erythromycin*, exhibited a strong inhibitory effect on all infections.

The effect of the chemotherapy drugs on the organs and cancer was evaluated with the O-Ring test and the following results were noted:
- *Methotrexate,* positive for the liver, thymus and for the cancerous breast and negative for the gall bladder, kidney and right breast;
- *Methotroxin* negative for the non-cancerous breast and positive for the center of the cancerous breast;
- *Fouracil*, negative for the liver, thymus, and cancerous breast and positive for the gall bladder, kidney and right breast;

- *Cytoxin*, negative for the liver, thymus and kidney, and positive for the gall bladder and both breasts.

Other anti-cancer substances she was not taking were evaluated by the same method:
- OH-1 was positive to left breast, right breast, liver and kidney;
- BCG-Waxin was positive to left breast, right breast, thymus and kidney (not approved in the US)
- mushroom was positive to cancer and all other body tissue;
- 1000mg vitamin C is negative to the cancer breast but at 500 mg positive for all bodily tissue;
- intrina DNA was positive to both breasts but negative for the liver;
- anti-oxida celgaard negative for cancer breast and liver and kidney;
- germanium is positive to both breasts, liver and kidney;
- beta-caratin positive to both breasts;
- garlic is negative to left breast and liver; carrot is positive to both breasts, and liver;
- whale meat is positive to the whole body;
- vitamin A , D, E tested separately is positive for the cancer breast;
- Substance P is negative for the cancerous breast and positive for the non-cancer breast:
- mycotatin is positive to cancerous breast but negative to the other breast.

Based on these results, the patient was given acupuncture to the neck to relieve the spasticity. She later developed chronic constipation. This may be due to the chemotherapy but we also noticed that the scar on her breast deviated from the normal large intestine pathway. (See figure 14 A-E) Acupuncture was given twice a year for several years and provided temporary relief. The patient lived in Oregon and did not have access to treatment in New York.

Eighteen years later, she was diagnosed with an acoustical neuroma in the lower middle right of the brain causing a loss of hearing, possibly explaining her inconsistency of instability in the neck by changing neck positions and the relationship to the thymus/thyroid being intermittent. She regularly has her neck treated with massage and chiropractic adjustments. Her constipation has resolved through self-monitoring. Four years after the diagnosis her neuroma is stable in 2008.

INFORMATION PROPAGATION WITH LASER

In the mid-eighties, Omura, with the assistance of Shinnick, conducted an examination of a patient. But instead of using a non-conducting probe with direct O-ring application, or a conducting probe with indirect O-ring, a laser beam was used as a probe to stimulate the stomach representation point (Ren 12) 中腕 zhongwan. This was done from a distance of about eight meters. Placing an aspirin in the vicinity of the beam caused the O-ring of the subject holding the laser pointer to open when the beam was targeting the Mu point for the stomach. Dr. Omura deducted that an 8 mm watt monochromatic concentrated beam (laser) positioned in the proximity of the control substance carries the molecular information to the subject to be examined at a distance. It is obvious that the practical applications of this indirect method are innumerable: from difficult patients to dangerous animals, the laser beam method could help make a diagnosis without the need to touch the subject, all the while maintaining a safe distance.[37, 38, 39, 22]

Many things are now possible thanks to the ORT, like finding an infection on an X-ray, MRI or CT-scan and determining the proper agent for treatment; or even determining anomalies in tissue samples.

MICROBIAL AGENT MIGRATION

In one case in 1986 Omura found the migration of helicobacter pylori from the stomach to the heart. He had suggested the involvement of helicobacter pylori in stomach ulcers and cancer before the scientific community accepted the concept and rewarded Australian doctors with the Nobel Prize for that discovery.

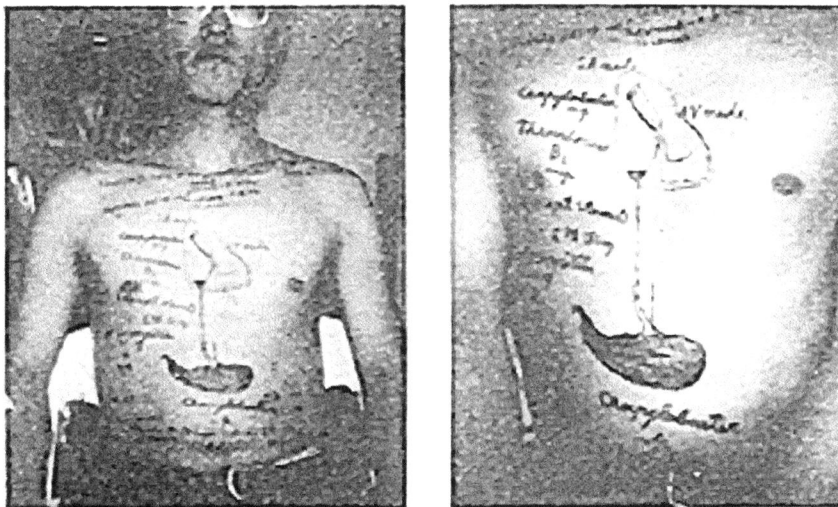

Figure 21
1986 Microbial agent migration [39A(p. 60)]
This figure is reproduced with special permission of Yoshiaki Omura, M.D.,Sc.D.

CHANGES IN BIOCHEMISTRY DUE TO PAIN

Using the O-ring, Dr. Omura was able to localize neurotransmitters and other substances present in areas affected with changes in microcirculation and pain. When the area tested positive for a microorganism, taking a matched anti-microbial agent before acupuncture decreased pain. [40]

In most cases acupuncture can relieve pain, but when it was unsuccessful Dr. Omura almost invariably detected the presence of bacteria, virus or fungus. He also observed that even using the right antibiotic was often not enough to relieve the patient's symptoms. By testing the affected area he soon realized that abnormal areas are always affected by poor blood circulation, therefore the antibiotic could not reach its target.

Through the ORT, one can perform a compatibility test for microbial agents with the right anti-microbial agent, i.e. the right antibiotics for a particular bacterium. Once a match is found, giving acupuncture locally 20 to 30 minutes after taking the antibiotic yields a much better result.

Acupuncture has a well-known effect of vaso-dilation at the level of the microcirculation, allowing the antibiotic to reach the affected area more quickly.

BIOCHEMICAL PRECURSORS TO CANCER AND CIRCULATION DISTURBANCES

Dr. Omura had an intuition early on about the importance of the blood flow in the area affected by pain, cancer or internal functional problems. He wrote in 1983:

"… And since any circulatory disturbance can (directly or indirectly) create pain, abnormal sensory function, muscle spasticity, muscle atrophy and many varieties of clinical symptoms, blood pressure and blood flow measurements at various parts of the body can be invaluable diagnostic tools, as well as a quantitative means of evaluating therapeutic effects. In fact, it is the author's belief that wherever there is an abnormality or a problem, there is also a corresponding circulatory disturbance." [40]

More recently he successfully used the ORT with Tromboxan-B2, a powerful vaso-constrictor, as the reference control substance to show that there is always a correlation with increased concentration of Tromboxan-B2 in a painful area, or an area affected with cancer or another functional problem. He also showed increased circulation from circulation disturbance by infusing paper with Qigong and placing the paper over the abnormal location. [41,42]

The research on the local sub-clinical infection prompted him to investigate the immune system and how infections of the thymus gland could affect its functioning and create an immune-deficiency syndrome. He then formulated the hypothesis that longstanding infection with the presence of heavy metal deposits and long exposure to EMF is a formula for cancer. He was able to demonstrate that if you have the right cancer marker (oncogen C-*Fos*), a certain neurotransmitter (acetylcholine), and a local hormone (*tromboxan B2*), you could reliably make a cancer diagnosis with the ORT. Because of his discovery there are now two schools of ORT for Physicians in Tokyo and his method has been adopted as an effective screening method in major Japanese hospitals. [43]

When all four co-factors are present, then special attention for cancer is required.
Four co-factors:
1. Increase in Oncogene C-fos AB2,
2. Marked increase in Intergrin $\alpha 5\beta 1$,
3. Disappearance of acetylcholine (Ach)
4. Marked increase in mercury (Hg) [44]

LONGEVITY

In the mid-nineties Dr. Omura became fascinated with longevity and visited Mrs. Calumet in France, at 121 she was the oldest living human on record at the time. He asked her the secret ingredients of her long life. She mentioned three things: Olive oil, a small glass of Port wine every day, and… Cheerfulness! He also estimated her telomere. Telomere is the molecular structure located at the end of the chromosome that controls the programmed death of the cell, also called apoptosis.

The amount of telomere decreases with age, therefore, infants have the highest amount and ultra-centenarians the lowest.

1998 Dr. Omura was able to estimate the amount of telomere in various age groups. This could potentially have an interesting application in forensic medicine and archeology. He also observed an intriguing phenomenon: after acupuncture on St 36 (a very important point in the classic Chinese meridian system), the amount of telomere increases considerably. Could it be that the ancient Chinese practitioners were right? In fact, one of the ancient point formulas for longevity includes St 36 (Zusanli足三里), Sp.6 (Sanyinjiao三阴交), and K.1. (Yongquan涌泉).

Another astounding fact was observed during the study of telomere levels. In cancer patients the amount of telomere in cancer tissues are always higher that the telomere of the normal tissue. Dr. Omura was concerned that giving acupuncture to cancer patients would increase the cancer telomere too, therefore increasing its growth. But to his surprise, when acupuncture was given to St 36, the cancer telomere was reduced to the normal value of the normal tissue, indicating the cancer replication was inhibited. [45]

EMF AFFECTS ON HUMAN'S BIOCHEMISTRY

Dr. Omura then started to look into environmental factors that could interfere with the therapies and discovered the effect of the EMF (Electro-Magnetic-Field) on the biological tissues and deposits of heavy metal as cofactors in the pathology he found.

In 1993 Dr. Omura published an article on the detrimental health effects of EMF. Using the ORT he was able to detect the appearance of several well-known cancer markers after exposure to the EMF generated by various common home appliances like TVs, computer screens, microwave ovens and cell phones. The presence of Thomboxane B2, Oncogene C-fos A 1 or 2, Integrin α-5 β1 in the areas exposed to EMF seemed to be related to the length of exposure and aggravated by the presence of deposits of heavy metals in the area. In the same article Dr. Omura reported changes in the stereoscopic structure of amino acids exposed to the microwave oven. He observed that most amino acids were converted from the normal L-form to a D-form and therefore could compromise the nutritional value of the food exposed to microwaves. This process could contribute to the development of cancer, Alzheimer's, and probably other diseases. [46]

Other independent researchers, who used the ORT in 2001 at the University of Istanbul, showed the correlation for the grip force, measured with a standard dynamometer, and ORT results when a group of people were exposed to facial expressions indicating crying or smiling.[47]

Exposure to a smiling expression increases the muscle strength while crying decreases it. Mrs. Calumet's ancient wisdom was confirmed!

In 2003 another independent researcher demonstrated the importance of ORT in managing a case with multiple hepatic abscesses. The patient had been treated unsuccessfully with three different antibiotics and the condition was deteriorating. With the use of ORT the pathogen was quickly identified and the drug compatibility test showed that two of the three antibiotics were ineffective, canceling the effect of the only effective one. Two different antibiotics were found to be compatible and effective, and the patient had an immediate clinical improvement. [48]

In the same year independent researchers published another article about a case of MRSA (methicillin resistant Staphylococcus Aureus) infection treated successfully with the administration of antibiotics and cilantro according to the ORT results. [49]

In 2003, using the ORT, L-Homocystine was found to be the most sensitive and reliable control marker for the screening of cardio-vascular diseases. [50]

CHAPTER SEVEN
SHINNICK'S CLINICAL
APPLICATION OF THE O-RING

Using the ORT on a regular basis I was starting to observe new and interesting pathways that were different from the Traditional Chinese Main Meridians System 中医主经络系统 zhongyi zhu jin-gluo xitong. Some of the new pathways appeared in a circular shape and I decided that it would be worth spend time investigating this phenomena. I needed to formulate a new theory based on the results of the ORT independently from the Chinese interpretation and knowledge of its classic energetic system. I chose to start an independent study to try to determine if there was an applicable clinical value of these findings.

This study was conducted at the Center for Sports and Osteopathic Medicine in New York from 1986-1991 with a patient pool of one hundred patients per day. Richard Bachrach, D.O., Steven Weiss D.O., and Mary Bano, D.O. evaluated the patients making an independent Western diagnosis of each patient while I evaluated and treated the patients based only on the ORT findings. Each week I prepared a clinical report of all the patients I had treated with a summary of the findings and the patient's progress. This report was given to Dr. Bachrach, the President of the Center. During the time of the study (1986-1991) every treatment was based only on the findings of the Bi-digital O-ring test method. Only after the study had ended did I have consultations with Drs. Bachrach, Weiss and Bano about the patient complaints, physical findings, and western medicine diagnoses and we tried to integrate them with the ORT findings. Adriano Borgna, M.D., L.Ac., and Jacob Heller, M.D. assisted Shinnick in many of the cases treated at the Center and Dr. Borgna, with the author's help, prepared Figures 6A and 6B, which were based on lectures by Omura. [3]

All the cases that will be presented in this chapter were photographed during the study but the quality, angles, and patient privacy precludes using those pictures. In order to illustrate our findings we used models as templates and superimposed pathways that were electronically cropped by a computer from the original pictures.

The patients, the physician, the acupuncturist and a witness signed informed consent forms. This form explained the procedure and the possible side effects of acupuncture according to New York State law at that time. See sample in Appendix A. It was a research protocol of the International College of Acupuncture and Electro-therapeutics. Also, the technique of the Bi-digital O-ring Test (Omura O-ring) was explained in an informed consent form signed by each patient. See Appendix I.

Most of the pathology seen at the Center for Sports and Osteopathic Medicine has to do with musculoskeletal pain. The ORT procedure was used to differentiate pain related to the dermatome caused by musculoskeletal injuries or from pain related to an internal organ and referred to the surface by its own meridian pathway. A pre-screening protocol technique was developed in order to quickly determine the health status of the patient and the origin of the pain by examining each vertebrae and Alarm Point (Organ Representations Point or Mu Point) for abnormality.

Based on the results of the ORT, abnormal Mu points and adjacent points belonging to the Urinary Bladder classic meridian 膀胱经 pangguang jing on the back were treated with acupuncture. In many cases I found abnormality just at the site of the vertebrae, sometimes the abnormal areas corresponded to a dermatome and in this case the acupuncture was performed along the abnormal area and on the tender points within that area. Sometimes the painful areas seem to have definite boundaries and did not seem related to a dermatome. In these cases the acupuncture was applied just to the boundaries found by the ORT. In the majority of cases acupuncture, performed following the finding of the ORT, was very successful in treating the pain; however between 5 to 10% of the 400 patients experienced only a temporary relief and had to come back for more treatments. In most of these cases the pain was related not to the local dermatome but to an internal organ and these are the cases that will be presented in this chapter.

The general principles of the BDORT (see Chapter 2) were applied to find abnormal areas and then a tray with the microscopic slides was used as reference substances to identify the organ involved. The slides were placed face down so that neither the patient nor I could read the label in order to achieve a sort of double blind method. Once a match was clearly found that slide would be used as a control substance to trace and image the abnormal pathway.

The advantage of using the organ representation is that one needs no sample of organ tissue. The disadvantage is that there are differences between the Mu point and organ tissue for the lung above the shoulder. The pathway goes to Mu point if the Mu is a control reference and, if using organ tissue, the pathway goes through the Mu point and moves up toward the cervical spine.

Organ Representation Points for the Mu and Shu points are presented as Figure 6. To avoid possible confusion between an abnormal vertebra and Shu Points, only Mu points were counted as organ abnormalities in this study.

As a result of the studies most of the results were concentrated in the mid thoracic, the hips and the legs.

THE PHENOMENON OF CIRCLES AND PATHWAYS: THE DEVELOPMENT BASED UPON THE EXTERNAL OBSERVATION OF THE O-RING.

In 1986 we illustrated the evidence for the existence of circles on the meridians or pathways (Figures 11A and B) through an experiment with lung tissue and tobacco as the control reference.[3] Later, colon and lung circles were found on the subjects' nose, the bottom of the feet, the hands, and ears. Acupuncture on the nose circles shrank the size of the circles to a dot. See Figures 22A and B.

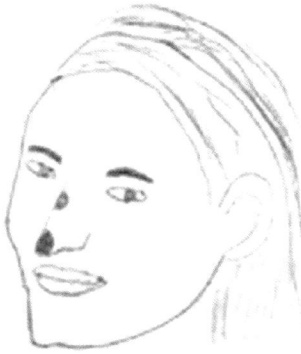

Figure 22A
1987 Colon (superior)
and Lung (inferior)

Figure 22B
A small dot appeared after acupuncture

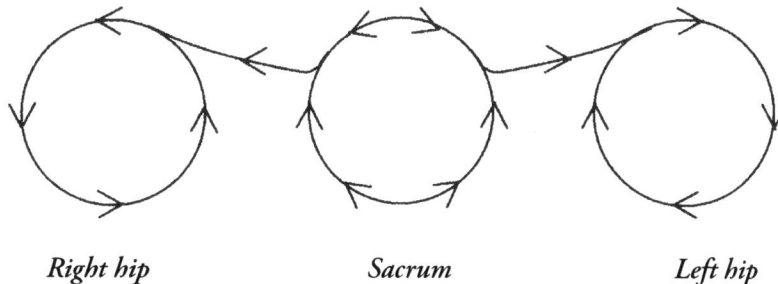

Right hip   *Sacrum*   *Left hip*

Figure 23

Many people wondered whether the pathway for the meridians ran along the fascia. Most were thinking of external fascia, but what about the inner fascia? In 1990, with the help of Joel Friedman, DDS, at the New York University Dental School anatomy laboratory, the inside of the viscera of a cadaver was moved aside so that the inside posterior fascia of the abdomen was exposed. An imaging was attempted using colon tissue. The results are shown in Figure 23 taken from a photograph after the imaging.

The circle is bi-directional, creating opposing directions from the same circle. From a third dimension, bi-directional implies spin. Each 180-degree turn changes direction as indicated in the linear drawing.

MULTIPLE PHASES: HEART AND DIAPHRAGM
HYPERACTIVITY OF THE HEART SHIFTS THE LINE OF ENERGY

In earlier studies (Figure 24 and 25) imaging of the hypertension of the heart and diaphragm of the heart showed phases. The case history of hypertension of the heart is as follows: In 1989 a patient complained of pain in his armpit, "...feels like my chest is being torn apart." with the physical findings of an angle of Lewis restriction and chronic costochrondritis. The diagnosis was hypertension and somatic dysfunction of the left hemithorax. The heart organ representation point, or Mu point, was abnormal. Heart tissue was used to image the pathway. Acupuncture was performed along the pathway (seen in Fig. 24A & 24B) and then it was imaged again using the BDORT with a microscopic slide of the heart muscle as a reference substance. See Phase two below Fig. 24C& 24 D. A second acupuncture along this new pathway resulted in phase three below Fig. 24 E.

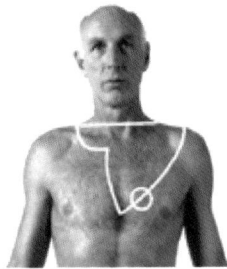

24A 4/89 Heart Phase one front

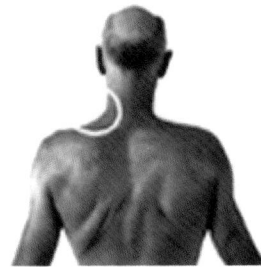

24B 4/89 Heart Phase one back

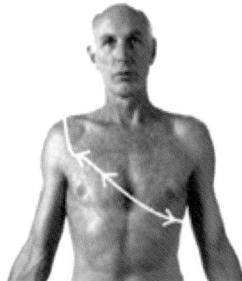

24C 4/89 Heart Phase two front after acupuncture

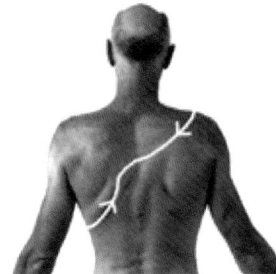

24D 4/89 Heart Phase two back

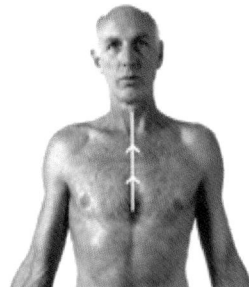

24E 4/89 heart Phase three after acupuncture

After three acupuncture treatments, a centerline appeared (Figure 24E), which came after the resolution of the aberrations due to hypertension and anxiety. In heart hypertension, the centerline seemed to rotate so that it goes around the body at an angle of 45 degrees as shown in 24C & D. From patient examination, it was found that this line corresponded to pain sensation with no pathology (he had a stress test for the heart) of the heart. But the important thing is that we were able to find a center pathway.

THE DIAPHRAGM AND ITS PHASES IN DIFFERENTIATION AND SYNCHRONIZATION

In 1989 a singer with cervical herniation complained of pain in her posterior deltoid and scapula, construction of her throat and breathing as well as chronic neck pain. Physical findings included a disc herniation C6-7, and disk bulging at C5-6. The diagnosis was intra-vertebral disc disease, cervical spine. A diaphragm tissue was used to image the pathway starting from the neck pain, seen as figure 25A 25F below. Starting from the xyphoid process the diaphragm splits in two directions.

Usually, if a toxin pathway was abnormal, such as the experiment with the lung using tobacco, it becomes normal after acupuncture. After needling the first pathway seen in fig 25A and 25B Phase Two appeared, in 25C. This went into Phase Three Fig 25E-F after a second acupuncture along the new pathway. And finally, after another acupuncture along the pathway, Phase Four appeared seen in Fig 25 G. Looking at the phases of the diaphragm, one can see the last position as being in the center of the body, presumable giving information bi-directionally.

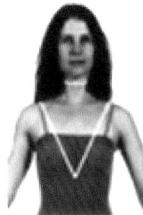

25A 2/89 Diaphragm
Front Phase One

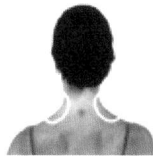

25B Diaphragm back
Back Phase One

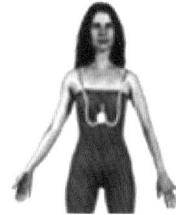

25C2/89 diaphragm
Phase two front

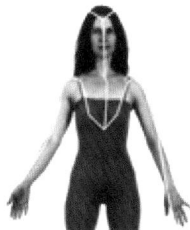

25E 2/89 diaphragm
Front Phase three

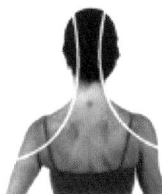

25F 2/89 diaphragm
Back Phase three

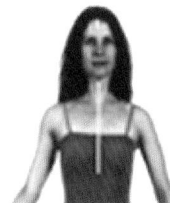

25G 2/89 Diaphragm
Front Phase four

This pathway changed according to the resolution of pain and tension. In these two cases the diaphragm pathway split (as will be shown in the triple warmer by Omura), and seemed to wrap around the shoulder and neck, causing pain and restriction in the throat. Like a neck noose hooked into the backsides of the neck and shoulder, it continued around the throat to the front of the neck, as shown above in 25A and 25B. The heart hypertension case was discussed earlier,

ORGAN AND TISSUE SAMPLES RELATED TO BODILY PATTERNS

Later clinical cases confirmed phase constriction in asthma, allergies, sinusitis, coughs, anxiety, deficiency and old age, as well as other lung diseases. In other words, each phase of the diaphragm has a pattern or phase which constricts respiration. In other cases one can see the relationship between muscle, tendon, joint, vertebrae and symptomatic pain patterns and body pathways related to organ and hormone derived tissue using the ORT test procedure. Structure misalignment is also associated with these patterns. The O-ring tests showed patterns of constriction in the thoracic and neck. Pain, constriction and entrapments of the hips, sacrum and legs are associated with certain organ patterns. For women these pain patterns are usually ovary derived. For men these constrictions are associated with the colon, bladder, prostate, gall bladder and testes. Below are a series of selected cases.

OVARY PATTERNS IMAGED OVER TIME 1987-1990

In 1987 a patient complained of constant pain to the left hip and medial calf. Western X-rays showed scoliosis to the left lumbar spine L3-4 and a 1.5 cm shorter left leg, pronation to left and a negative bone scan. The diagnosis was tendonitis in the left hip, tibialis porticos, and subtalar joint dysfunction. After the usual procedure, the hip pain returned again and again. Acupuncture treatment gave only temporary results. Starting from the hip pain area, the point was stimulated with a piece of tape, and microscopic organ slides and other samples of tissue were placed face down in the vicinity of the patient. Using the direct BDORT, therefore using the patient fingers and with her free hand positioned just above the microscopic slides, through a process of elimination the ovary tissue was found to match the abnormal pathway with the strongest response. The imaging is shown in Figure 26 A-J. Seven separate patterns of abnormal pathways mappings were demonstrated using the ovary tissue from 1987 to 1990 on this same patient. Using this technique, the patient got longer pain relief but it was never resolved completely. Acupuncture was performed along the pathway and on the tender points. Later on, in 1991, a cyst was found on her ovary and excised. In 1997 she still had some pain but was able to go through the rehabilitation training for strength, which previously had always triggered a pain reaction. Now her condition could be managed with less treatment, which was mostly physical therapy.

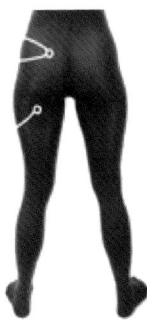

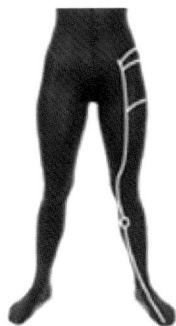

26A 12/7/87 Ovary   26B 12/7/87 Ovary   26C 5/26/88 Ovary   26D 9/26/88 Ovary

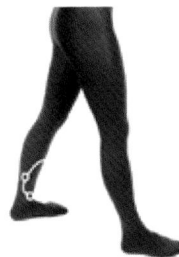

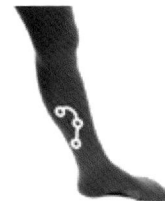

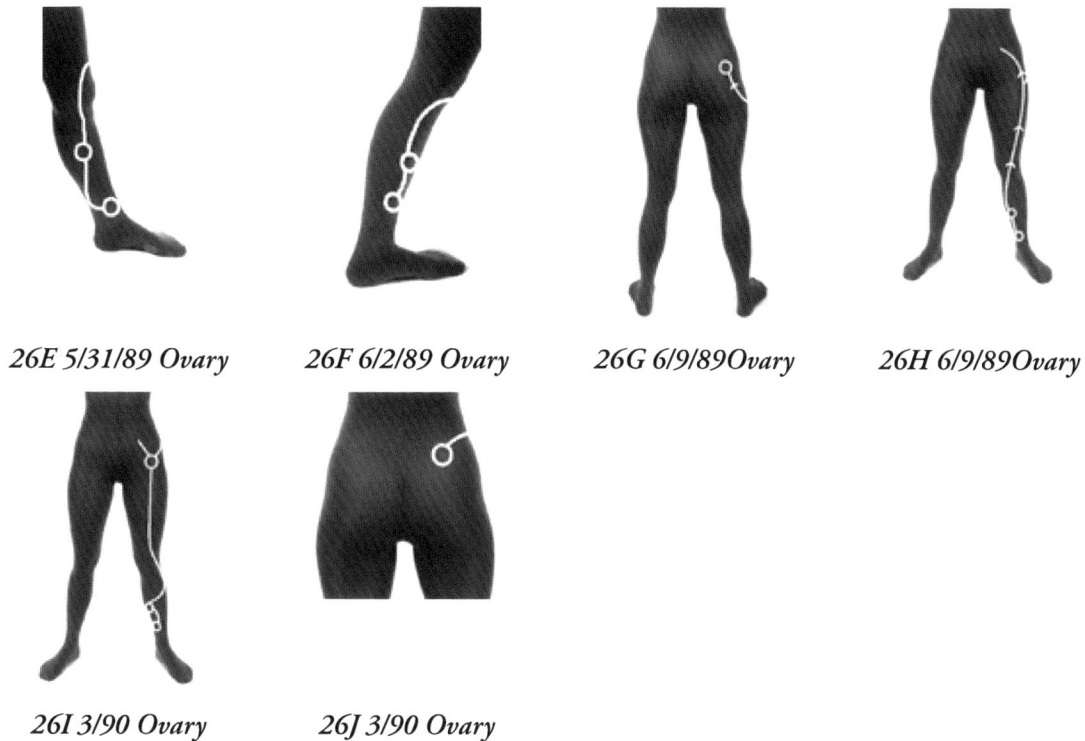

26E 5/31/89 Ovary   *26F 6/2/89 Ovary*   *26G 6/9/89Ovary*   *26H 6/9/89Ovary*

26I 3/90 Ovary   *26J 3/90 Ovary*

In 1989 another ovary pathway was found in a patient who complained of left sacral pain and left radiculopathy, with physical findings of postural imbalance and psoas insufficiency. The diagnosis was somatic dysfunction SI left. Based upon the previous case, ovary tissue was tested with the BDORT on the painful area and it led to the imaging on Fig. 27.

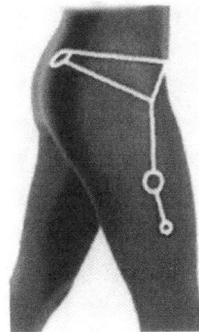

Figure 27 1989 Ovary Pathway

Several similar other cases are shown in Figures 28-31. Figure 28 resulted from a patient complaining of pain to the sacrum and the abdomen. Eight years earlier she had fractured her sacrum in a soccer injury; the diagnosis was somatic dysfunction of the SI. Laboratory tests showed dysphasia of the cervix. A microscopic slide of cervix dysplasia was used as a reference substance in this case. This is shown in the pictures below. Two months later she suffered a spontaneously ruptured ovarian cyst. Two years later Figure 28C and 28D reflect her pathways. The pathway of 28C and 28D appears to encircle the umbilicus. By observing the pathological pathway in picture 28 A and B it is a reflection of the hip and leg pain this patient was experiencing.

28A 9/89 Dysphasia of Cervix   *28B 9/89 Dysphasia of Cervix*   *28C 10/91 Dysphasia of Cervix*   *28D 10/91 Dysphasia of Cervix*

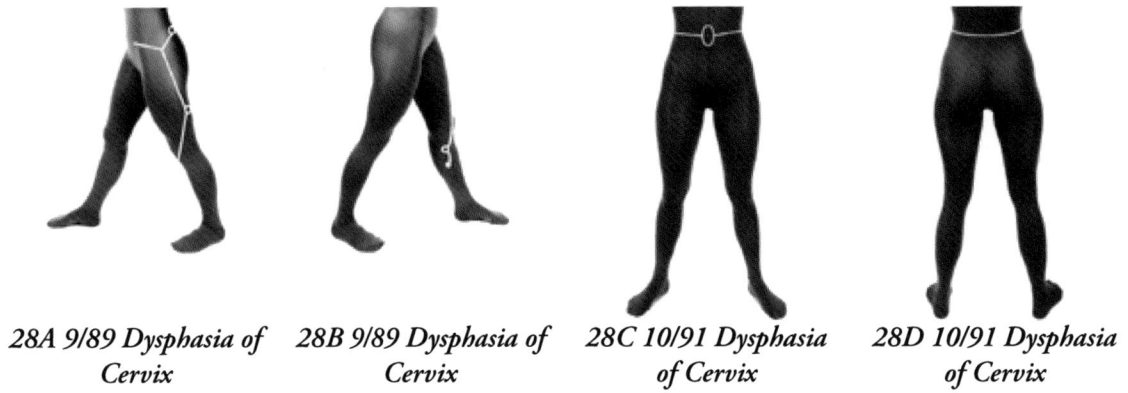

Another patient complained of pain to her medial calf. Physical findings included pronation of both feet and obesity. An ovary tissue was used for the BDORT imaging and it is shown below in Figure 29.

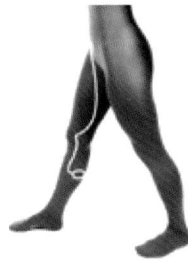

Figure 29 1989 Ovary

In 1989 a patient complained of pain in the hip. Her physical findings included depression and outbreaks of herpes every time she was under stress. The diagnosis was chronic immune deficiency. Because of previous experiences the ovary tissue was used again as a reference substance for the BDORT and you can see the pathological pathways in Figure 30 A and B.

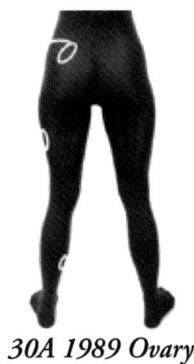

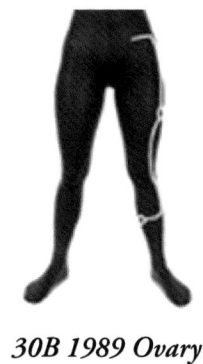

30A 1989 Ovary   *30B 1989 Ovary*

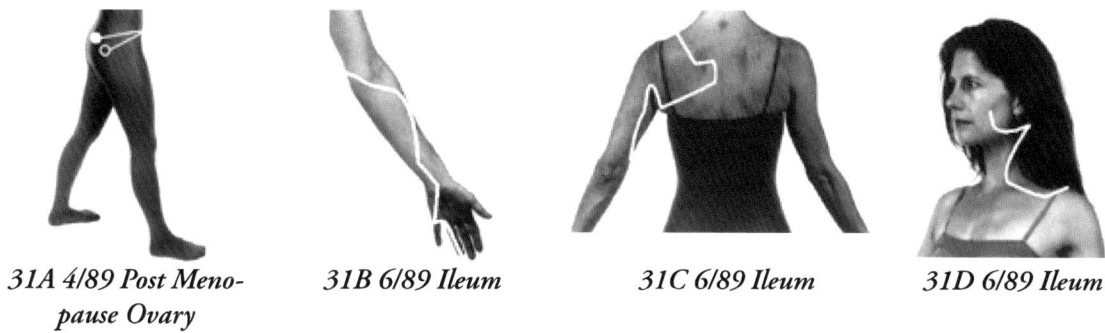

| *31A 4/89 Post Meno-pause Ovary* | *31B 6/89 Ileum* | *31C 6/89 Ileum* | *31D 6/89 Ileum* |

During the same year a 73-year-old patient complained of neck and hip pain. Physical findings included a left posterior neck lymphoma, left atrophy of trapeziums, cervical side bend limitation. X-rays showed bone density loss, anterior vertebral osteophytes and hip restriction of side bend. The diagnosis was disk disease, degeneration of the lumbrosacral spine, somatic dysfunction of the cervical spine, arthritis, and osteoporosis. Having tested the patient with a large number of microscopic slides a positive response was found with a postmenopausal ovary tissue and the pathway detected can be seen in Figure 31 A. Superior patterns of pain relate to ileum tissue 31 B-D.

IMPLICATIONS OF THE OMURA THYMUS NETWORK
AND SHINNICK OVARY PATHWAY TO WOMEN'S HEALTH

After examining Omura's thymus network with the female images as a general understanding, I intended to see if this was useful with clinical cases. Case 8 and 8A show the picture of the Omura thymus network using thymus tissue as the control reference. Over the years we started to see a number of patients with breast cancer. We started to notice by using the BDORT that women with breast cancer often had thymus network blockage, spasticity, cervical problems, or other structural problems with the shoulder, neck, and upper thoracic. The treatments were focused on normalizing spasticity to the chest, neck and shoulders. For the women with breast cancer or tumors, examination showed blockage to the areas indicated in the Omura network pattern, on the axilla, pectoralis muscles, and cervical asymmetry dysfunction, particularly at the exit of the third cervical nerve under the mandible around the sternocleomasatiod muscle, and at the second and third thoracic vertebra around the paravertebral muscles. Manual pressure on the spastic muscle seem to be able to normalize the thymus and mammary glands pathways

Several cases of infertility were treated successfully by needling the pathways found with the BDORT using the Ovary tissue as the reference substance. Most of these patients presented with hip and leg pain.

MALE PATIENTS WITH ABNORMAL ORGAN
PATHWAYS TO THE HIP AND LEGS

A male patient presented with low back and feet pain with cramping. Physical findings from an MRI showed herniation at L4-5, decreased mobility of the ankle joints, slight scoliosis left, mild narrowing of L4-5, L5-S1 spaces, a 14 mm pelvic tilt, asymmetrical transitional vertebral (between

T-12 and L-1) obesity, mucous colitis proctitis, and radiculopathy right or pain down the right side. The diagnosis was somatic dysfunction of the lumbar spine. The sacral area with pain could be mapped with the BDORT by using a microscopic slide of human testes, shown below, and two weeks later we mapped both the colon and testes using a germanium diode for direction (diodes travel only in one direction) in Figures 32 A-E.

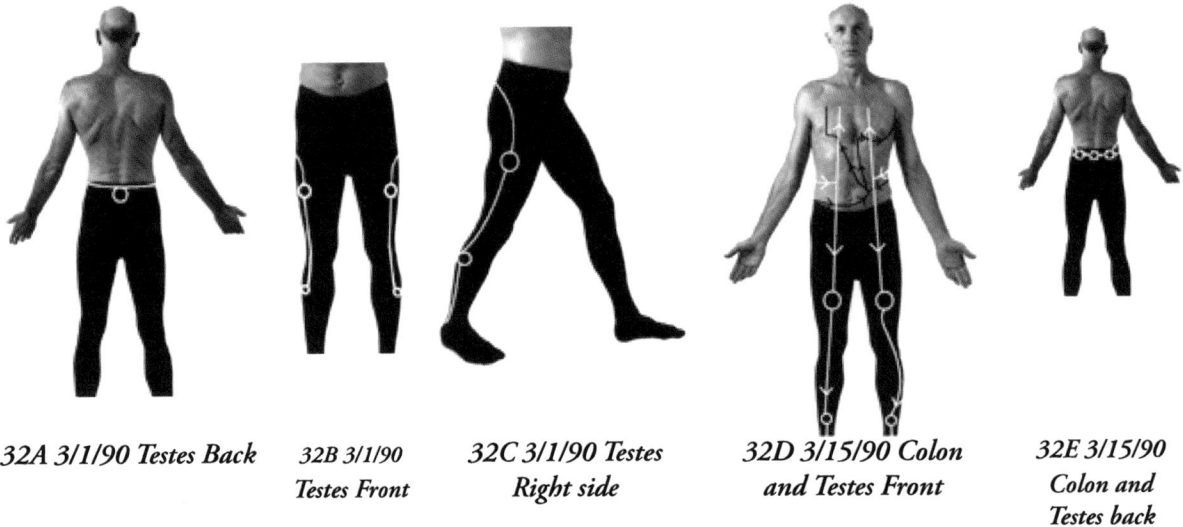

| *32A 3/1/90 Testes Back* | *32B 3/1/90 Testes Front* | *32C 3/1/90 Testes Right side* | *32D 3/15/90 Colon and Testes Front* | *32E 3/15/90 Colon and Testes back* |

Germanium diode specifications manufactured by NYE (177), PRV 200V Max Vf -1.0V @100mA, If = 160mA, Ifrm - 250 mA, trr-50 ns. New-Tone Electronics, Broomfield, NJ 07003

Another male patient complained of constant pain to his right hip and the physical findings included scoliosis to right lumbar, large osteophytes L1-5, moderate narrowing L4/L5/S1, right femoral head 2 cm lower, right iliac crest 1.5 cm lower, right hip spur. The diagnosis was hip pain due to psoas insufficiency, chronic disc disease L4/5.

The usual method to detect a possible reference substance with the BDORT (testing samples until one that is compatible is found) revealed that the microscopic slide of pancreas tissue had the strongest response. The pathways imaged with the pancreas tissue are shown in Fig. 33 A-B. The patient's foods and drinks were also tested using the painful area as the reference control with the BDORT and it was found that Gin had a strong negative response. The patient stopped drinking Gin and with the needling along the pathway imaged with the pancreas tissue slide the pain was completely relieved to the point that he started to take figure skating lessons at age 45. One year later the pain came back and this time the BDORT revealed that the strongest response was obtained by a microscopic slide of gallbladder. He admitted of often having outburst of anger so he was taught a breathing technique and with few treatments of acupuncture he had complete relief.

| *33A 3/88 Pancreas* | *33B 3/88 Pancreas* | *33C 6/88 Gall Bladder* | *33D 6/88 Gall Bladder* | *33E 6/89 Testes* |

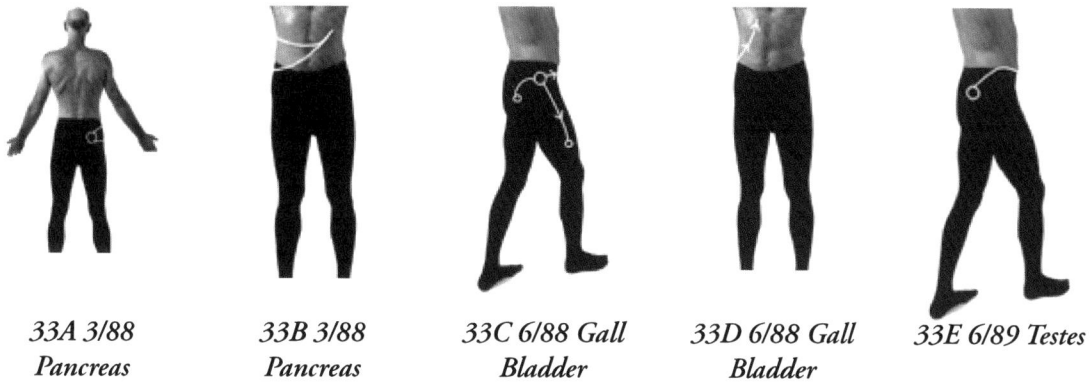

In 1989 a patient presented with back pain, and an MRI showed a large herniation at L4-5 and compression on his thecal sac, with sacroiliac joint radiculopathy. The diagnosis was somatic dysfunction of the lumbrosacral spine, and psoas insufficiency syndrome. The organ representation point for gall bladder was abnormal and Figure 34 A and B reflects imaging from this point.

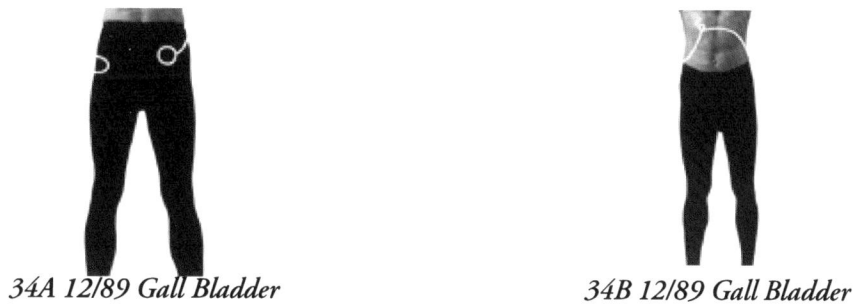

| *34A 12/89 Gall Bladder* | *34B 12/89 Gall Bladder* |

In 1989 a patient complained of chronic right hip pain aggravated by gardening. Physical findings found chronic constipation; an MRI showed L5-S-1 disc herniation and L4-5 bulging. The diagnosis was somatic dysfunction, lumbrosacral spine. In this case the BDORT revealed that the microscopic slide of colon tissue had the strongest response associated with the painful area and the pathways are shown in Fig. 35

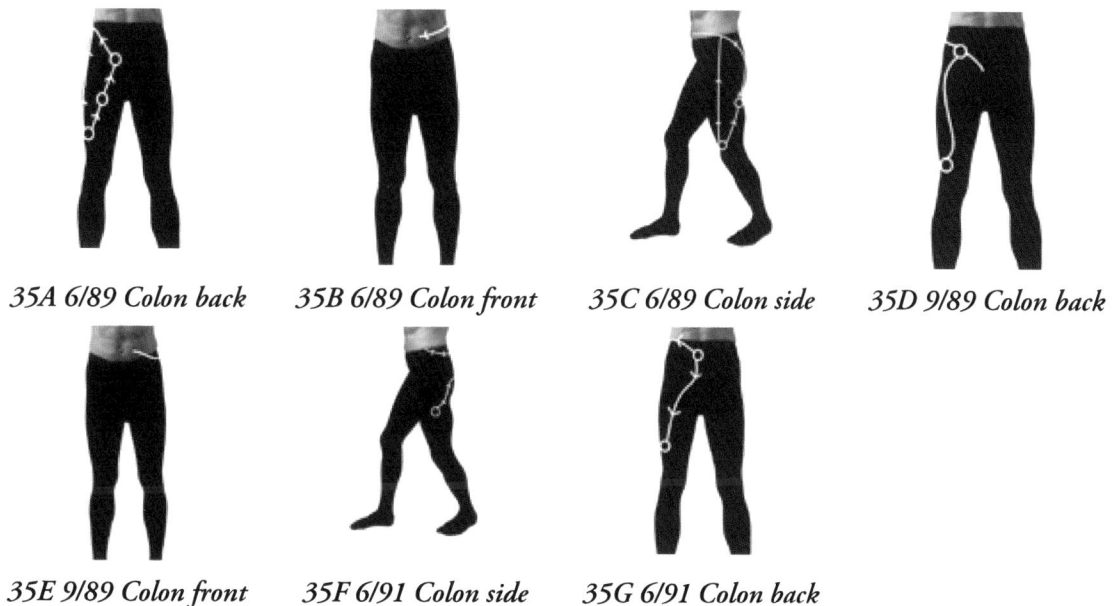

| *35A 6/89 Colon back* | *35B 6/89 Colon front* | *35C 6/89 Colon side* | *35D 9/89 Colon back* |

| *35E 9/89 Colon front* | *35F 6/91 Colon side* | *35G 6/91 Colon back* |

49

In 1988 a patient complained of constant pain in both hips. Physical findings included right thoracic scoliosis, weak abdominals and moderate narrowing of L-5. The diagnosis was chronic immune deficiency and psoas insufficiency. In this case a microscopic slide of the urinary bladder had the strongest response with the BDORT. Figure 36 below shows the pathological pathway. Two months later I was able to successfully map the pathway from the hip pain points without using the urinary bladder tissue. In other words without tissue, using the BDORT, the bladder pattern could be found from the pain area.

Then, using bladder tissue, another imaged pathway was found. This is shown below in Figure 36A. When acupuncturing the bladder pathway from the tissue it remained stationary. But, when the pathway imaged without bladder tissue was acupunctured, it moved to the pathway imaged with tissue. Figure36B. The imaged pathway without tissue is a pain pathway, deviating from the tissue imaged bladder pathway. With treatment it fuses with the bladder pathway, although the Traditional Chinese bladder pathway goes down the back of the leg and sacrum.

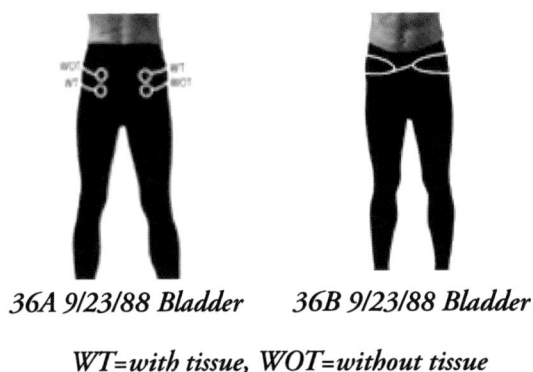

36A 9/23/88 Bladder   36B 9/23/88 Bladder

WT=with tissue, WOT=without tissue

LONGITUDINAL ENTANGLEMENTS THROUGH TIME

In 1987 a patient complained of chronic pain to his right hip, radiating downward. Physical findings showed right thoracic scoliosis 38 degrees and anterior spondylolisthesis at L3, L4, L5. The diagnosis was tendonitis of the right hip. He described the pain as if two snakes were wound tight around his leg, with intense pain upon arising in the morning, lasting for up to one hour. Using a Doppler flow meter and ankle cuff I measured the venous pressure on the pedal artery and found it to be low, so he was instructed to "bicycle" in bed with his legs up over his heart to facilitate venous pressure before he got out of bed. The intense early morning pain disappeared. As usual, through the BDORT I found the tissue with the strongest response to the hip pain point, which was compatible to bladder and prostate tissue. These two pathways were imaged on separate occasions and are compared to each other.

Mapping of the area with the two tissues was performed and it is shown in Fig. 37. More sophisticated medical analysis was performed on his bladder by his physician and a sphincter problem was diagnosed. Medication was prescribed and a majority of his symptoms resolved. He was later diagnosed with prostatitis.

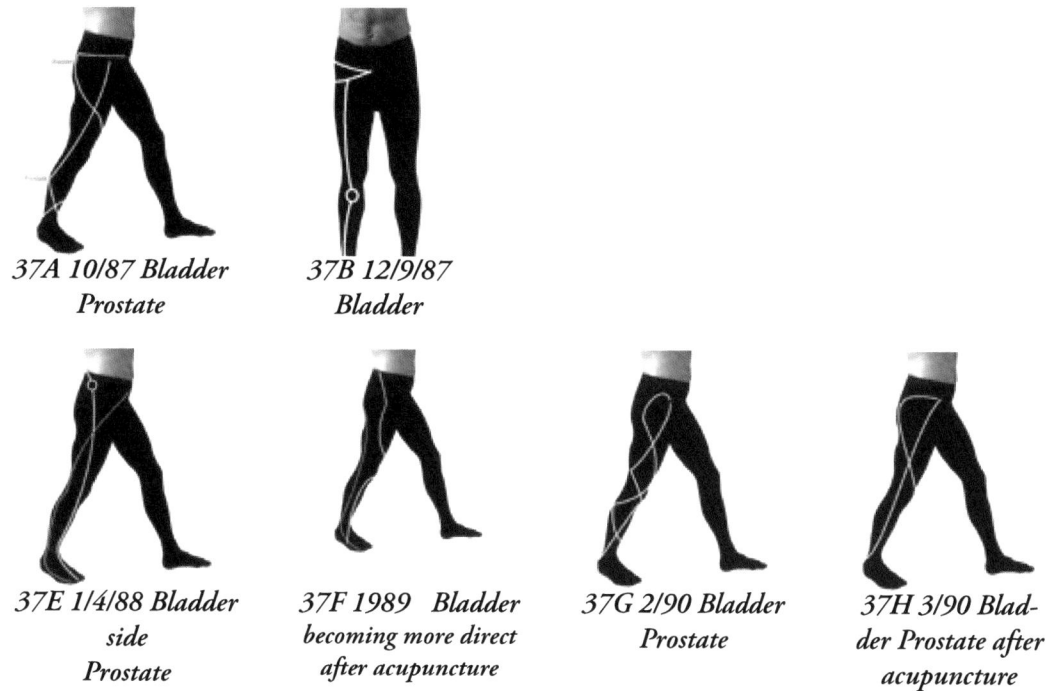

37A 10/87 Bladder
Prostate

37B 12/9/87
Bladder

37E 1/4/88 Bladder
side
Prostate

37F 1989   Bladder
becoming more direct
after acupuncture

37G 2/90 Bladder
Prostate

37H 3/90 Blad-
der Prostate after
acupuncture

PATIENT WITH TWO CIRCLES
IMAGED BY SHINNICK WITH ACUPUNCTURE ON 7/9/88

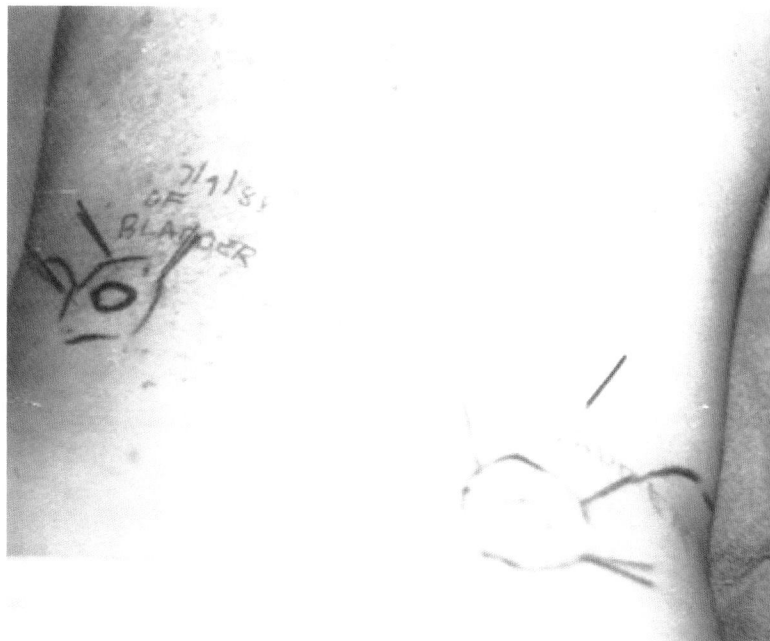

Figure 38

This patient was a professional racquetball player who suffered from back pains and this pattern emerged intermittently for a year, aggravated by depression.

SUMMARY: IMPLICATIONS

These unusual cases showed meridian patterns connecting the abdomen to the hip area with organ tissue matches for the colon, small intestine, gall bladder, pancreas, bladder and ovary. A spherical hollow shape was imaged at the posterior hip area of the pathway in all but one case. In all extra pathways the direction of the flow was always toward the organ (using a diode.) In the cases of colon, testis and ovary, multiple pathways and spheres were found. For the ovary and colon, these extended down the ilio-tibial band to the medial calf with the pathway direction going down then up on another branch toward the organ. Pathways were imaged randomly for diaphragm, ileum, jejunum, duodenum, thyroid, anus, Purkinje fiber, prostate, and heart. The diaphragm and heart were imaged in multiple phases after acupuncture. Patients with certain symptoms such as asthma or hypertension appeared under one phase, thus indicating locked patterns manifest in multiple locations on the body. Acupuncture has been shown to be effective in moving patterns to other locations after being stuck in certain phases. Scars along the pathway or internal pathology to the organ can cause the pathway to deviate. The largest association to these abnormal pathways was scoliosis, or asymmetry. A case with a confirmed bladder sphincter dysfunction and prostatitis resulted in a criss-crossing of pathways in the leg in three places over a three-year period.

These experiments and clinical cases show a moving energy pattern after treatment and a system of circles generating directionality that change with treatment. It demonstrated a resolution from bi-directional to unidirectional in the heart and diaphragm. In 24D the directions goes against each other in heart hypertension. This has implications for organ disease for pain patterns on the hip, sacrum and legs. In other words, pain in the hip, sacrum and legs can be organ dysfunction. In women these pain patterns can mean low or abnormal ovary production or dysfunction associated with spasticity, and pain to legs and hip. In men certain alcohols can have a bad effect on an organ or emotional outbursts, can create pain patterns in the hip and leg.

CHAPTER EIGHT
CIRCLES BEFORE AND AFTER STIMULATION ACCORDING TO OMURA

In 1989 Dr. Omura published an analysis of the circles and meridians and this chapter summarizes that article. With the O-ring Omura observed the transformation process with bio-chemical reactions in both painful and non-painful areas. Omura was able to detect "acetylcholine, serotonin, methionine-enkephalin, beta-endorphin, ACTH, secretin, cholecystrokinin, norepinephrine, and GABA within the entire area of the acupuncture points and their meridians, regardless of which meridian was examined." High concentrations of methionine-enkephalin, beta-endorphin, serotonin, and GABA were found in the traditional Chinese meridians, while ProstaglandinE1, dopamine, dynorphin 1-13, and VIP were found at the center midline of the meridian but not inside or outside the boundary of the acupuncture point. [30] However there were exceptions. In some individuals serotonin and other neurotransmitters such as GABA were found only in the meridian and not in the acupuncture points. Atrial natriuretic peptide was found in the heart meridian and its acupuncture points, gastrin was found in the stomach meridian and its acupuncture points, and testosterone and estrogen were found in the triple burner meridians and its acupuncture points. The substances found above in the meridians and acupucnture points were not found outside the meridian. Substance P as well as thromboxone B2 and L-tryptophan was only found in painful areas, but it was quickly changed into serotonin after acupuncture and pain relief.

When acupuncture was performed, atrial natriuertic peptide rapidly appeared and spread out over the body and then disappeared in twenty minutes; Acetylcholine and prostaglandinE1 appeared rapidly all over the body and disappeared in 4 minutes then reappeared only on the acupuncture point; Methionine-enkephalin spread out to the surrounding tissue outside of the acupuncture point, disappeared in 10-15 minutes and then reappeared in the entire area within the boundary of the acupuncture point. During the appearance of the above neurotransmitters (atrial natriuretic peptide, acethylcholine, prostaglandinE1, and Methionine-enkephalin) in the area just outside of the acupuncture point, (almost) none of these neurotransmitters could be found within the boundary, with the exception of the center line of the acupuncture point where the meridian was located.

While Dr. Omura was researching and testing the neurotransmitters relationship with the acupuncture points and meridians, he found a new pathway for the triple-burner meridian; he could trace it bi-laterally from the shoulders down to the testes or ovaries and back up to the shoulders.

Omura tested the meridians and acupuncture points after acupuncture, electrical stimulation at low frequency, mechanical pressure, soft laser with milliwatt output, and Qigong. Generally, the effect from acupuncture was the same as mechanical stimulation if the stimulation equaled 5 kilograms/cm_2 for ten seconds. It was the same with soft laser and electrical stimulation, but with Qigong the circles showed a slightly different behavior. The effect of Qigong transformed the circle in a doughnut shape as indicated in Figure 39 below. Note that with Qigong treatment most of the neurotransmitters have a unique distribution of "doughnut shaped" positive areas, but no neurotransmitters were found in the "hole of the doughnut," except in the center mid-line where the meridian was located. Omura also noticed that, when performing acupuncture, if needling was performed too far away from the center of the acupuncture point the previously observed effects would not occur to the same degree as when the acupuncture needle was placed near the center of it. As you moved away from the center — up to 7mm, you need to stimulate the needle or use electrical stimulation for some minutes to produce the same effect as when needling the center of the acupuncture point.

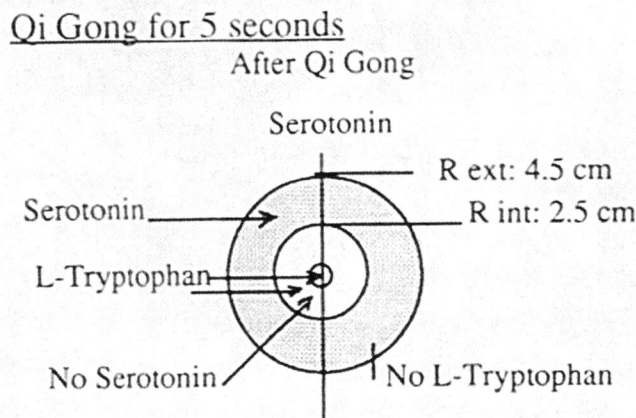

Figure 39 [30(p. 174)]
This figure is reproduced with special permission of Yoshiaki Omura, M.D.,Sc.D.

Figure 39 illustrates the effects of the application of external Qigong for 5 seconds from the index finger of the Qigong practitioner to the acupuncture points Ht.7 (about 8 mm diameter at the left wrist of a 30 year old, apparently healthy, white female volunteer) on the release of neurotransmitters and hormones. However, norepinephrine was the exception not shown here. Other neurotransmitters and hormones are Acetylcholine, PGE1, and atrial natriuretic peptide. They appeared rapidly all over the body and disappeared within 4 minutes. When serotonin does not exist in the acupuncture point or in the area surrounding the point, L-Tryptophan (which is the precursor of serotonin, see figure one) replaces it, with the exception of the centerline of the acupuncture point where the meridian is located.

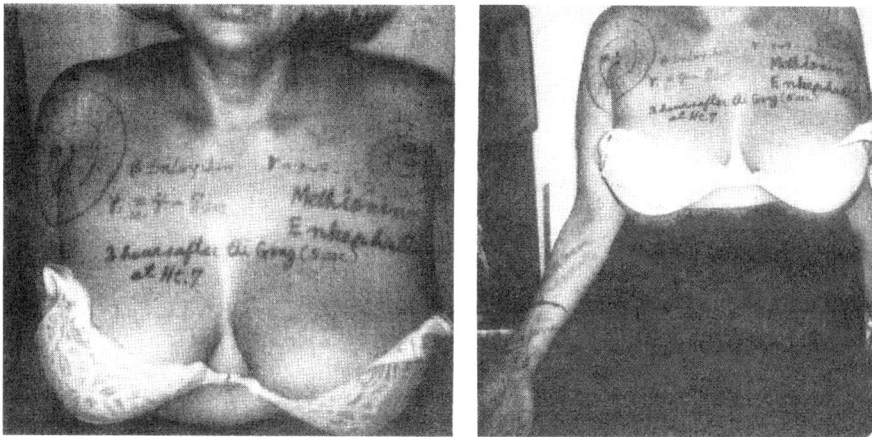

Note the doughnut-like shape of the circle on her shoulder three hours after Qigong on her heart in Figure 40. In Traditional Chinese Medicine, the first heart point is on the axilla, but with Omura's imaging he clearly shows that Heart 1 jiguan is superior to the traditional understanding. Omura's Heart 1 is in a form like Figure 39. In the center of the doughnut-like shape there is a smaller circle that has methionine-enkephalin in it but it doesn't appear anywhere else except at this point and the meridian line. Dopamine was also found in the doughnut-shaped area, about 4.3 cm from the center acupuncture point, but not in the doughnut hole, except the center point and meridian. Dynorphin 1-13   appeared in the doughnut shaped area with a radius of 9.2 cm and there was a high concentration of atrial natriuretic peptide in the center heart meridian acupuncture point. The doughnut hole also had serotonin but no L-Trytophan. VIP was found in the doughnut shape but not in the center or doughnut hole.

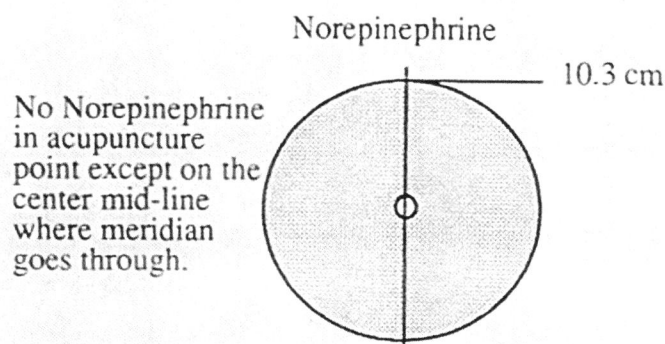

Figure 41 is a case where norepinephrine was found only at the center point of the acupuncture point and meridian line by Omura.

These figures are just samples of Omura's imagings for circles and represent the general structure and changes to the circle.

CHAPTER NINE
THE HUI HYPOTHESIS:
ACCUMULATED EVIDENCE

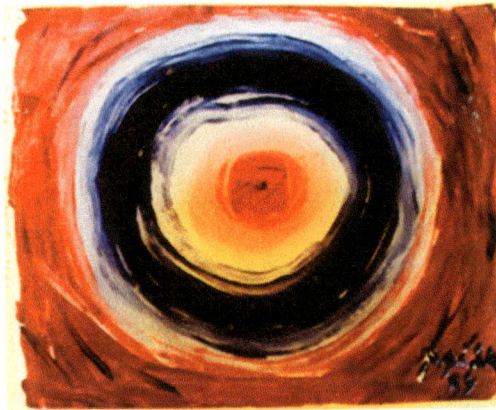

1984 Shinnick Painting
Aggregate of separate sequential time phases
All paintings in this Chapter, and front and back cover, are created by Shinnick

It became evident that a hypothesis had to be formed from the circles seen by both Shinnick and Omura, varying in location and organ system. In 1988 Shinnick proposed the Hui[1] hypothesis in an attempt to explain the accumulated evidence using the O-ring body surface imaging method, resulting in larger circles rather than small acupuncture points.   See Phase 1 next page.

The basic idea is that the inside of the circle inverts to the outside and the outside to the inside. As an example, the color red is inside the circle and black is on the outside. The opposite color serves as a background: i.e. inside, red dots with a black background and outside, black dots with red background. There is no solid color; it is a vibration field of opposites.

---

1 Hui means circle in Chinese. The modern Chinese character for circle is a square line within a square line; not too long ago the character was a circle in a circle, and the ancient character for circle was a spiral, taken from a whirlpool.

THE HUI HYPOTHESIS: A GENERAL THEORY

The Hui hypothesis is based upon the idea that the circle undergoes a reversal to the opposite; the inside of the circle goes to the outside and the outside of the circle goes inside. In the first phase the boundary separating the red inside and the black outside of the circle has a diffuse boundary as opposed to a distinct boundary. In the second phase the movement is inward, creating a circle within a circle. The inner circle still has red on the inside (with black background) and, outside the two circles, black (with background of red). In the third phase, there is a return to the configuration of the second phase, but now it is black on the inside (with red background) and red outside of the outer circle (with black background). The movement is outward. The space between the two circles is nondescript. This whole process is very fast. Phase 4 is like Phase 1 but opposite. This transformation takes about one second to go through its phases.

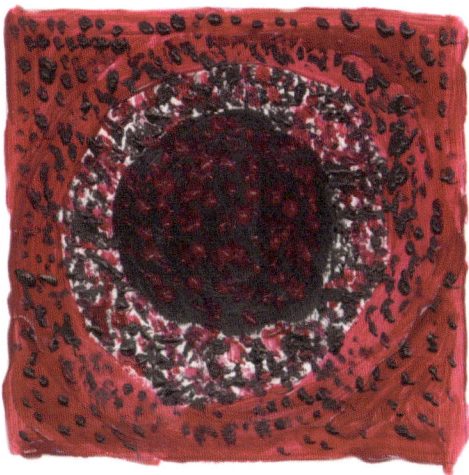

Phase 1

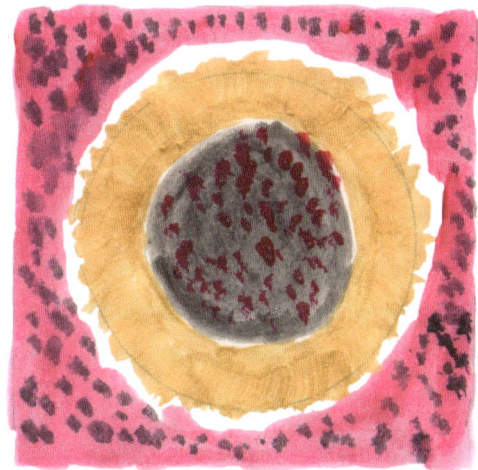

Phase 2

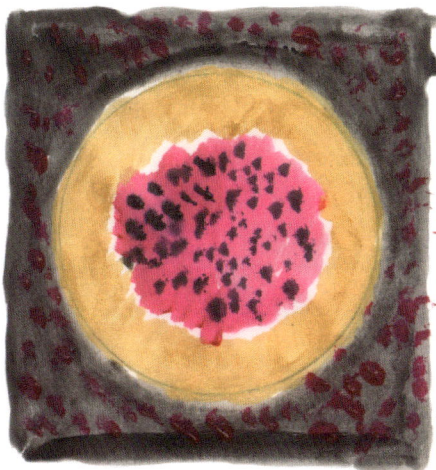

Phase 3

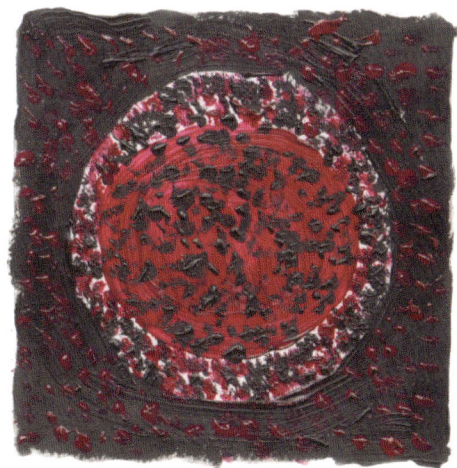

Phase 4

PARTICULARITY

The original hypothesis had six phases and this order was often confounding and not clearly understood. In order to clarify this hypothesis the current presentation was developed. Between Phase 1 and Phase 2 another phase appears periodically that is a distinct circle with an illuminated boundary. Here the inside and the outside are the same. This sub-phase is quick, like a camera flash, distinctly different from the sequential changes of the other four phases, called the Circle of Transformation (Phase 1.1), which causes a change from a vibratory to a stable field; this can be seen as a move from vibratory movement to a combined directional linear transverse movement within a distinct boundary circular form. Within the distinct circle is a stable field, creating the possibility for directional movement through the differentiated circle. Picture will follow as Phase 1.1, explained later.

Another sub-phase appears between Phases 2 and 3, Phase 2.1, a single point or nothing. There is a movement inward of Phase 1 and 2 to a point, Phase 2.1; then an expansion outward to Phases 3 and 4. The movement inward is a spin, the movement outward is a spin in the opposite direction. (In terms of healing one could look at this as inward internal healing and outward external healing, as in Qigong.) Outside the single point of Phase 2.1, the area is all the same, and when there is no point, the whole area has no form, it becomes a clear color blue (Phase 2.2), green (Phase 2.3) or yellow (Phase 2.4), or a fusion between dark and light, which will be depicted as a white state for current purposes (Phase 2.5). The explanation will follow after the four phases are discussed.

PHASE 1 CHARACTERISTICS

In Phase 1, the diffuse boundary, with distinct inner and outer differences, is the start and becomes its opposite, i.e., with black on the inside and red on the outside and with the opposite color as a background. This whole process starts again until it goes back to the beginning of Phase 1. More time is spent in Phase 1, with the diffuse boundary juxtaposed with the contrast of the inner and outer circles. The whole field vibrates as the small particles move positions continuously. The evidence of the difference between the inside and outside areas can be seen in the 1986 Figure 11, the triple blind study by Shinnick, Blumenthal and Berger. (The circle width is the width of the probe, and the boundary becomes distinct through imaging. The width of the circle is not as important as a boundary between different substances or polarity.) In this 1986 imaging, tobacco was used with the lung as the control reference, and it showed a difference between the compositions of the inside to the outside of the circle. This can also be seen in Shinnick Figure 22A, an imaging of an umunculus on the nose for colon and lung. This again shows a difference between the inside and outside circle. After stimulation the circle goes inward to a point, which will be discussed in Phase 2.1. Figure 31A of a post-menopause ovary on the hip of a patient with osteoporosis shows the difference inside and outside the circle. However, after acupuncture the circle shifted to another location and did not display the difference between inside and outside.

Omura showed in Figure 41 that the inside of the circle is different from the outside with no norepinephrine inside and norepinephrine outside. However, he found norepinephrine at a small center point in the circle. He also showed that after outside stimulation the size of the circle diminishes like Phase 2.1. In the thymus network, Figure 8, Omura showed circles with the inside and outside different. One can see that Omura's Norepinephrine (1989) or the Shinnick toxic lung circle (1986) have differences between the inside and the outside. Another example is Omura's Serotonin circle of 1989, which shows Serotonin on the inside with L-Tryptophan on the outside, which is not shown.

HUI HYPOTHESUS

Circles not to scale   Yes means compatible with control substance and no
means no response to control substance i.e. lung, ovary or Norepinephrine.

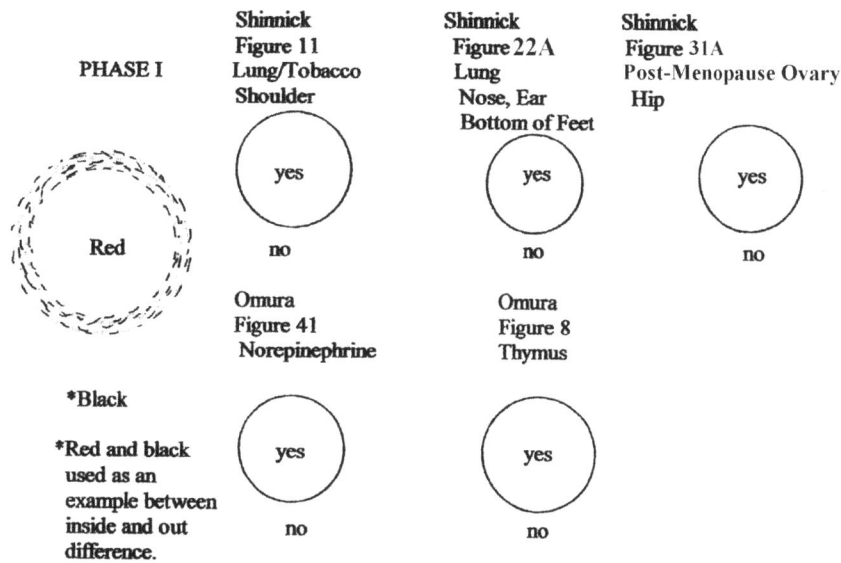

PHASE I	Shinnick Figure 11 Lung/Tobacco Shoulder	Shinnick Figure 22A Lung Nose, Ear Bottom of Feet	Shinnick Figure 31A Post-Menopause Ovary Hip
Red	yes / no	yes / no	yes / no

	Omura Figure 41 Norepinephrine	Omura Figure 8 Thymus
*Black *Red and black used as an example between inside and out difference.	yes / no	yes / no

PHASE 2 CHARACTERISTICS

Phase 2 of the Hui hypothesis is a doughnut-like ring with the inside of the doughnut different from the outside. The doughnut-like ring is nondescript and luminous. Figure 38 for the bladder shows the circle as a doughnut-like shape. In the 1989 Figure 39 Omura found a doughnut-like shape on the heart meridian after Qi Gong was administered, confirming aspects of the Hui hypothesis with a difference from the inside of the doughnut to the outside.[51]

HUI HYPOTHESIS

Circles not to scale.

PHASE 2

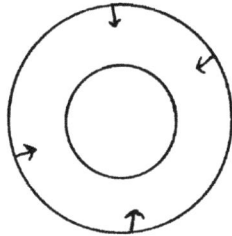

| Shinnick Figure 38 Bladder Superior to Iliac crest of hip | Omura Figure 39 Heart Ulnar wrist | Omura Figure 41 Heart Inferior deltoid, lateral pectoralis |

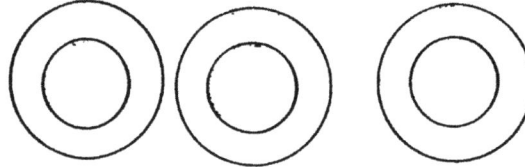

This can also be seen in Omura Figure 41 after Qigong. In Omura's 1989 imaging of the heart, observation shows a contraction of the circle into a doughnut-like shape, which he found after 5 seconds of Qigong. So there is evidence that this double circle appears after some Qigong, but it also appears independent of treatment.

HUI HYPOTHESIS

PHASE 3

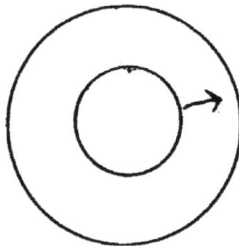

| Shinnick Figure 33C Gall Bladder Hip Outward | Shinnick Figure 33A Pancreas Hip Outward | Shinnick Figure 35C Colon Quadriceps Outward | Shinnick Figure 35G Colon Sacrum Outward |

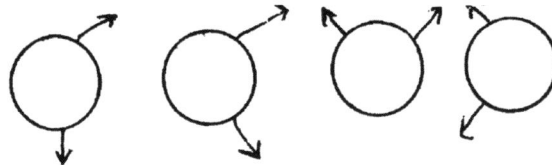

PHASE 3 CHARACTERISTICS

Phase 3 of the Hui hypothesis goes back to the configuration of Phase 2, but opposite, it goes outward. This phenomenon is dealt with above in the experimental observations. The directionality can be seen in Figure 33A, 33C, and D; Figure 35C, F, and G; and Figure 24C going outward. Figure 33C and 33A also show this outward movement in more than one angle. From clinical observation it appears that the circles were in the expansion mode. This is seen in clinical patients who report pain or dysfunction of some sort, usually an injury to the spine or a joint.

PHASE 4 CHARACTERISTICS

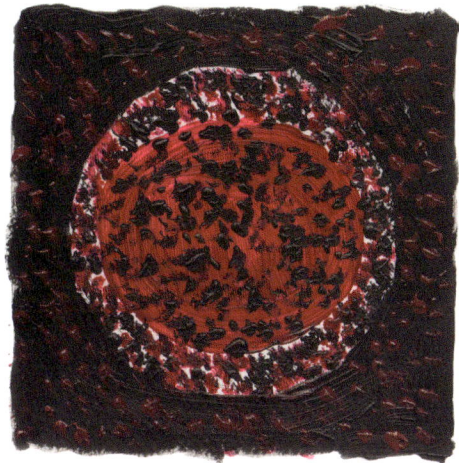

Phase 4

Phase 4 is like Phase 1 except there is a reversal and the process starts over again until it comes back to Phase 1. Omura has shown that after acupuncture the inside L-tryptophen and outside serotonin reverse; what is inside goes to the outside or vice versa.

CIRCLE OF TRANSFORMATION: ABRUPT AND INSTANTANEOUS

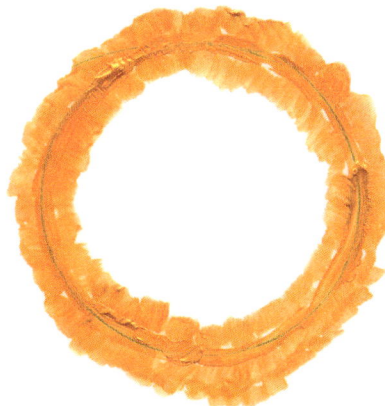

Phase 1.1

Phase 1.1 comes right after Phase 1 and is very quick, like a camera flash, and is in sequence but of another order. This distinct quick movement (moving outward and inward) is illuminated with a gold ring or illuminated boundary replacing the diffuse boundary of the red and black. When this happens, both the inside and outside are the same, non-descript and hued with gold. Outside forces can transform this into circular movement.

Shinnick's imaging in Figures 32A-E of the testes on the medial ilio-tibial band, on the lateral superior soleus, on the medial quadriceps on L4 and L5 of the lumbar spine, on the spinous process, and on the iliac crest shows circles with the inside and outside the same. Also, Shinnick imaged the inside fascia of the abdominal cavity in Figure 23, which had the inside of the circles the same as the outside. In the ovary imaging (cyst on the ovary), Figure 26, the inside and outside were the same and the circles persisted over time but moved locations. Also dysphasia of the cervix in Figure 28 again shows a shifting of the circles over time but retaining the same characteristics. Figure 31 of the ovary shows the same characteristic. In Figures 33-37 for the pancreas, bladder, and colon, it shows the same characteristics with no difference between the inside and outside. Force from above and below would force the circle to go around in a bi-directional way, spinning off into two lateral circles, as happened in the colon imaging on the sacrum (Figure 32E), and shown also in the internal fascia of the abdomen (Figure 23). In Figure 23, the directionality of the circle is bi-directional, and the following diagram tries to explain how that happens by adding assumed forces which could explain this.

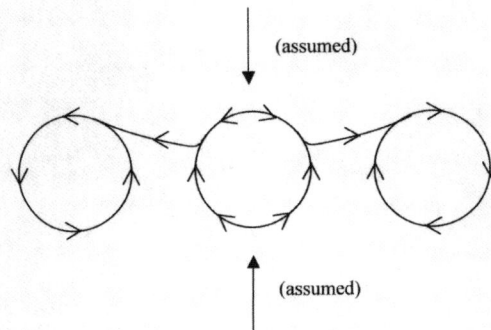

HUI HYPOTHESIS

These circles are not to scale. For Phase 1.1 the inside and outside are the same and the movement is out and in at the same time, or bi-directional, perhaphs spinning. The distinct ring is gold which leaves a hue over both inside and outside so as to make them the same. The control substance is after the figure number and the location on the body is indicated.

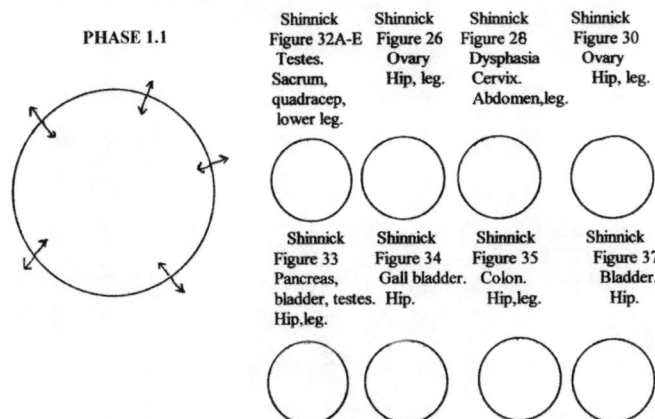

There are imagings of upward and downward motions, as for example in Figure 33C of the gall bladder and quadriceps, and 35F and G with the colon and hamstring in a downward movement. Figure 32D of the testes has an upward and downward movement. Figure 25G shows upward center movement in the diaphragm after acupuncture as does the heart in Figure 24E on the sternum medial center. So there is evidence of upward movement in the center and downward movement laterally.

CIRCLE OF TRANSFORMATION: EQUATORIAL MOVEMENT

Phase 1.2

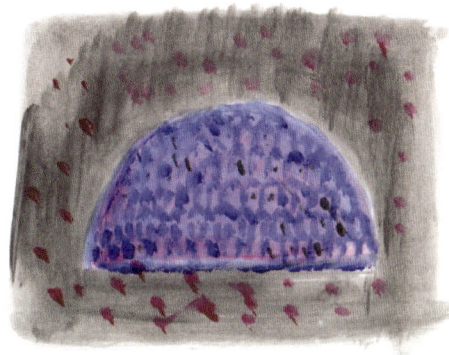

Phase 1.25
Third Dimension

The rapid circle ring illumination triggers another phenomenon, an escape from the vibratory displacement of opposites sequence. The ring of transformation is periodic; the inside of the ever-inverting circle becomes clear blue inside. It is like a camera lens clicking. A third dimension shows that it rises above the surface of the body and has a dome-like shell structure of hexagons. The dome is made up of lines joined in hexagonal structures in such a way that the individual hexagons together make a circle that expands and contracts. The blue hexagon dome creates the illusion of clear blue, but this is the hexagons emanating a blue light that appears as a blue hue, creating the possibility of permeating the inside from the outside and vice versa. This is created by the expansion of the circle up from the surface of the body like a dome in the third dimension with red on the inside of the dome and black on the outside. The domed hexagons create an illusion of pure color but are like a lattice between the inside and outside. This is the coupling of linear into curvature. It can expand up into a dome or down into a point. See discussion later.

Omura showed that the acupuncture point of Stomach 36 penetrates below the deepest layer of the tibialis anterior muscle, deep into the body of a cadaver, about 1.8cm wide and 1mm deep.[52] If the circle has a dimension below, then symmetrically it will occupy space above. The clear opening at the center of the circle has no experimental evidence to confirm this through this body imaging technique, but it appears that it may open to another dimension outside the body (or possibly another way for the body to communicate, without linear movement, to itself). Allegorically, there is a stillness inside the circle much like field transmission (rather than linear); instantaneous, communicating inside and outside the body. This would be a static, stabilized state accessing another dimension or simply communicating outside to inside the body (or vice versa). The last phase of the diaphragm (see Figure 25G) showed an up and down line, and perhaps when things resolve in the total organism and the body is at rest or in a lower energy state, the movement of the circle stops. In this state information is transmitted not linearly but instantaneously throughout the body. Other dimensions could be discussed.

LATERAL TRANSVERSE MOVEMENT

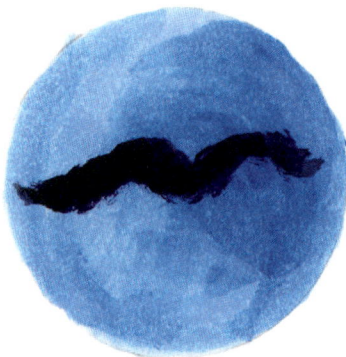

Phase 1.3

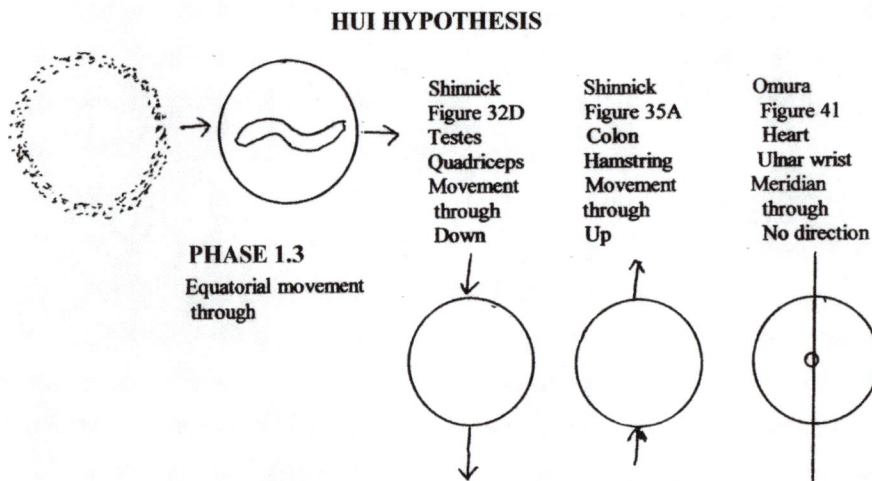

HUI HYPOTHESIS

PHASE 1.3
Equatorial movement through

| Shinnick Figure 32D Testes Quadriceps Movement through Down | Shinnick Figure 35A Colon Hamstring Movement through Up | Omura Figure 41 Heart Ulnar wrist Meridian through No direction |

In the lateral movement, a distinct purple amount (quantum), like a drifting cloud, comes across the clear inside circle dissects the circle and is gone. It is not continuous but a distinct amount, more or less the size of the circle's diameter and with a width of about one fifth of the circle, it appears as if riding a wind, or, pushed by some force. Relative to the vibrational energy, it moves slower. One can see that Shinnick Figure 32D has a downward movement using testes tissue as a control reference on the quadriceps. Shinnick Figure 35A shows upward movement using colon tissue as a control reference on the hamstring. Omura shows this in all of his diagrams where the centerline of the meridian transects the circle. Omura Figure 41 shows equilateral dissecting of the circle with the inside and outside different. Omura did not use a diode to determine direction but one assumes it moves one way or the other. In the Shinnick figures the inside and outside images are the same but nevertheless it shows a movement through. Experimental imaging supports this idea. The drifting of the cloud like a stratus formation could be just one direction of force, like a spurt, or an organ in transition from one state to another, i.e. digestion to non-digestion, or liver, heart, intestine phase changes. In other words, catching a spurt or movement through would be hard for the O-ring which just gives one aspect of the process. Figure 31A shows a circle with a center that is different, like phase 1.2 where the changes are equivalent to Phase 1.1 after acupuncture.

CHARACTERISTICS OF BLOCKED LATERAL MOVEMENT AND A DIVERSION TO ANOTHER DIMENSION (SPIN OUTWARD OR SPIN INWARD)

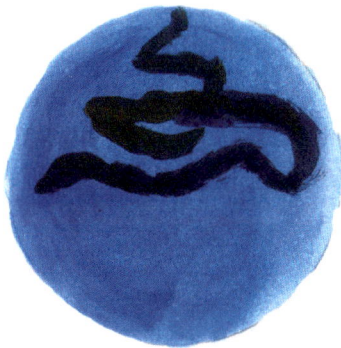

Phase 1.31

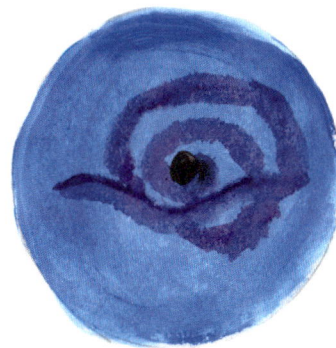

Phase 1.32

There are three possibilities in Phase 1.31. The first is that the change in direction goes to a Z-axis to the third dimension as shown in Fig. 1.25. Another is a change in direction on a two dimensional level as shown as a shift from A to C after B is blocked, as shown in Figure 13. An experiment was conducted on a meridian line, which was blocked with a diode (one side goes in, the other side is blocked) and showed a change in direction (A to C). This experiment was done because it was noticed that with a toxic substance to the lung, tobacco, the meridian deviated and the diode was used to mimic this behavior. The third is a change in direction where X=0, Y=0 and Z=0 and the direction change goes to the middle as a point, as shown below in 2.1.

PHASE 2.1 MOVEMENT INWARD TO A POINT, SPIN INWARD (HYPERCYCLE)

Phase 2.1

HUI HYPOTHESIS

| PHASE 2.1 | Shinnick Figure 22B Colon Ear, nose, bottom of feet | Shinnick Figure 31A Post menopause ovary Hip | Omura Acupuncture circles from 3 mm to 2.7 cm shrinking to one half size after acupuncture. |

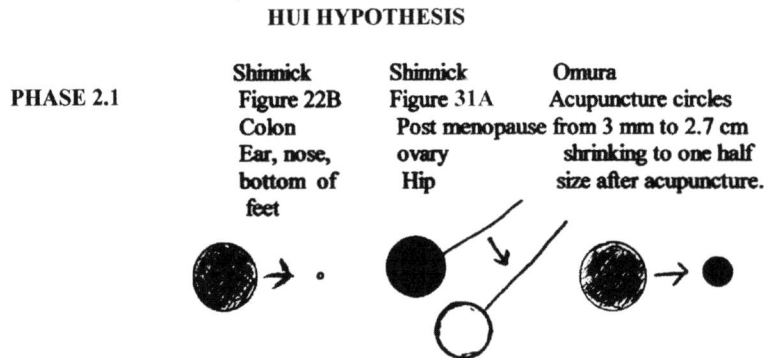

Phase 2.1 is like Phase 1.3 with movement through the center of the circle, a stratus-like cloud drifting across the center to the other side, then it turns upon itself (like being blocked) and starts spinning inside the circle like a cyclone or dragon, with the tail up and the head going into another dimension and then is gone. The spin inward goes to a dot and the spin outward goes out and is gone. One can see this in the third dimension shown above; however, this change of direction can be to another side of the circle beyond the equator if it is not totally blocked. Or this can be into the center where the three axes are 0. This can be seen in 22B after acupuncture to the umunculus of the colon and lung on the nose; the same phenomenon also existed for the ear and the bottom of feet. You can see above in Figure 31A that the circle (inside different from outside) shifts so that nothing is under the acupuncture point since it moved locations going Phase 1.2 to 1.1, reversing the process. Omura showed how the circle shrinks after acupuncture.[53]

HUI HYPOTHESIS: PHASES 2.2–2.5

Phase 2.2

Phase 2.3

Phase 2.4

Phase 2.5

The flushing, as shown in Phases 2.2, 2.3, 2.4, and 2.5, on occasion becomes either blue, yellow, green, or no distinct color (a fusion of dark and light across the whole circle). A clear color appears, as if painting over the pattern with a color with no form. It looks still even though it seems to drift across. The circle became obscure. The order of these things is not necessarily in the order presented, only at different intervals of the circle transformation. One should note that an imaging through the O-ring seems to catch a glimpse of the dominant time spent in a phase.

Omura shows that the triple warmer (esteriol/estridal and testoserone), stomach (gastrin), heart (atrial natriuretic peptide), and norepinephrine are released throughout the body after acupuncture. (See beginning of Chapter 8,) One would assume that these substances are periodically emitted from the organs for a more global response.

The phase of the flushing effect is a global response. We've discussed stimulation and global responses from patients. There can be another aspect to a global response and that is when the inside/outside of the body unite for a moment which overrides the particular circle transformation and its effects. In other words, there is a unity with the body and the universe, with particularities, like the pathway system, vanishing. A differentiation has to be made between a global versus a particular locality. Patients have reported this flushing or movement of energy all over their body after acupuncture. The global response could be seen as a synchronization of the individual to the vibration of the earth and this is blue. The flushing comes when the body acts as a single unit rather than being differentiation.

The aperture opening of a clear color is also when an organism is at rest, the stratus cloud when energy comes from one direction, the spinning when many forces are at work. All of these are possible influences on the circle, which in this regard is an acupuncture energy point. The colors can be different organ energy resolution to full permeability and movement throughout the body, having its own dynamic in the biochemistry of transformation as shown by Omura.

One thing seems obvious, that things are not static in the human organism, and it is subject to many forces inside and out, which happen all the time, and the dominance of one force or the opposing of forces creates changes in the Domonal. Or, perniciously, an external pathogen, i.e. bacterium, virus, parasite, or fungus, can capture the energy of an organ and piggyback on an existing network, moving within the circle or to another location.

There are also possibilities to send internally generated fields of energy to outside the body and also resonance to the vibration of the earth through synchronization of body energy through self-care practices.

This clear blue global response is periodic and is known through the teachings of the Medicine Buddha and Sidha Yoga blue pearl. This should be seen in terms of non-locality of the circle as it opens to space and out of uni-dimensional time, engulfing an organism.

A NON-EQUILIBRIUM STATE IN THE ORGANISM

Prigogine shows a similar configuration as Phase II in the nucleation of liquid droplets in super-saturated vapor.[54]

When the circle is smaller than the critical size then you see a movement out like the one shown in Phase III. If the circle is larger than the critical size then the movement will be inward as shown in Phase II. If there are fluctuations, boundaries will dominate as shown in Phase II and the fluctuations regress.

Prigogine shows how opposing forces function when the circle has movement around it as shown above and this is a more stable situation.[55] The diagrams of Prigogine start with the assumption of a non-equilibrium state and the clinical evidence from the O-ring imaging shows that acupuncture circles are far from in a constant equilibrium state as is taught in Traditional Chinese Medicine but are in constant fluctuation. These forces from within and without determine the size of the circle, the configuration, and the directionality, which can be outward.

Prigogine presented a circle as a non-equilibrium situation with the spinning a resolution of one force acting on another. Equilibrium is a fiction in the human organism. We are far from an equilibrium condition caused by psychic behavior, weather, and the unstable conditions of life. It is therefore tempting to suggest that the origin of life may be related to successive instabilities somewhat analogous to the successive bifurcation that has led to a state of matter of increasing coherence.

SHINNICK SUMMARY

In the International Chinese Medicine paradigm, organs have pathways on the surface of the body flowing in a linear fashion according to the time of day. In addition, the Triple Warmer is a pathway which regulates heat in the body throughout the upper, middle and lower aspects of the body. Omura showed the adrenal gland is the gland which images the pericardium while the ovaries and testes image the Triple Warmer. There are brother and sister pathways with one more dominant than the other. Evidence has been brought forth to generally prove such a system. The O-ring is a technique which makes it possible to image these organ pathways on the surface of the body, which Omura and I, working independently, have shown through publications during the last several decades through the O-ring. However, this evidence shows differences from the Traditional interpretation.

In the mid-1980s I decided to create a triple blind study of the method. This was done by the direct method with a subject's fingers, with the subject and operator not observing what imaging a third person did with a non-conducting probe. We randomly attempted to image the lung pathway coupled with a known toxin to the organ, tobacco. This pathway deviated from the normal one and showed spheres that were different on the inside and from the outside. Later stimulation to this aberrant pathway caused it to shift approximate to the traditional pathway. A larger study needed to be conducted to interpret this understanding. This 300 case study with independent diagnosis by three physicians resulted in only 10% of pain patients not able to resolve the pain by electro-therapy and acupuncture using a standard protocol of testing each vertebrae and organ *mu* points on the front of the body and stimulating the dermatome of the abnormal vertebrae and resulting abnormal organ. The dermatome is the area lateral to the vertebrae which is innervated by the spinal nerves exiting the vertebrae. Of the thirty cases not resolved by this technique, random organ samples or other tissue was tested for compatibility to pathways imaged. The confounding results showed an assortment of pathways and circles not typical of the Traditional Chinese Theory. Omura also produced results which in certain regards showed similarities. The acupuncture points were larger, changed shape and location after stimulation and, as Omura showed, had an assortment of organ bio-chemical substances on the pathways and circles. Inside the circle was different than outside in substances and polarity, however, instances showed inside and outside the same with distinct boundary spheres. Stimulation changed all of this. Other tissue showed pathways such as the diaphragm, bacteria, dysplasia of the cervix, ovary and testes.

In the 1980s I presented the Hui Hypothesis to explain these confounding evidences. The essence of the Hui Hypothesis is that the circles are constantly changing by inverting, from inside to outside in four phases. These circles are vibrating in constant flux in fields that differ from the outside to inside with diffuse boundaries. The O-ring test reflects a dominant phase of the circle. The phases move through changes constantly over the course of seconds but have dominant phases with distinctly different patterns. Two additional phases were added to the original four phases fifteen years later to account for evidence not fitting into those first four. Images show an inclusive field inside the circle and outside (Phase 1.1) the boundary is different from the inside and outside. When this happens, transverse linear movement can happen or be deviated from a direct route to the other side. Experiments proved this. This deviation can change angles or go up and out or down into the body, or simply concentrate to a point.

Evidence also shows double circles through both my images and Omura's reflected in Phase 2 or 3 of the Hui hypothesis. Phase 2 which has distinct boundaries collapsing in, while Phase 3 moves out. Clinical imaging supports this. At times there is a spinning of the linear movement around itself to a point or disappears to another location, or a flushing as indicated in Phases 2.2 to 2.5 as evidenced by Omura's bio-chemical reaction which spread over the whole body for a time. Patient's also report a flushing feeling after acupuncture stimulation. External Qigong influences this process in distinct ways, as Omura found. In Qigong, a Master can emanate energy from their hand to another. Also a person can direct Qigong emanation inward to their own body which is called internal Qigong.

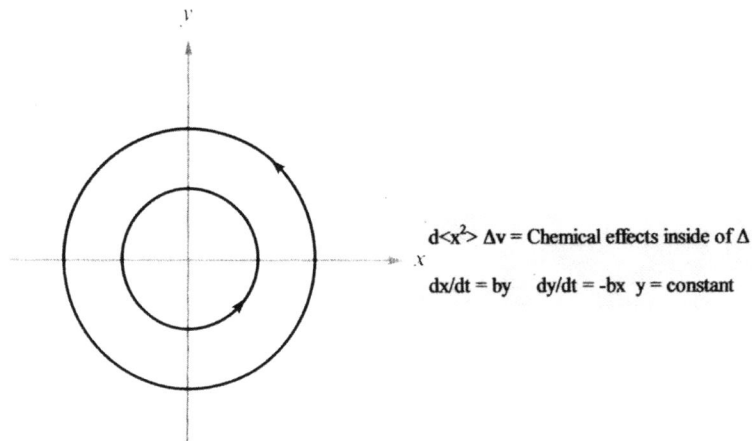

$$d\langle x^2 \rangle \, \Delta v = \text{Chemical effects inside of } \Delta$$

$$dx/dt = by \quad dy/dt = -bx \quad y = \text{constant}$$

$$X = 0$$
$$Y = 0$$

$$dx/dt = by$$

$$dy/dt = bx$$

Hypercycle

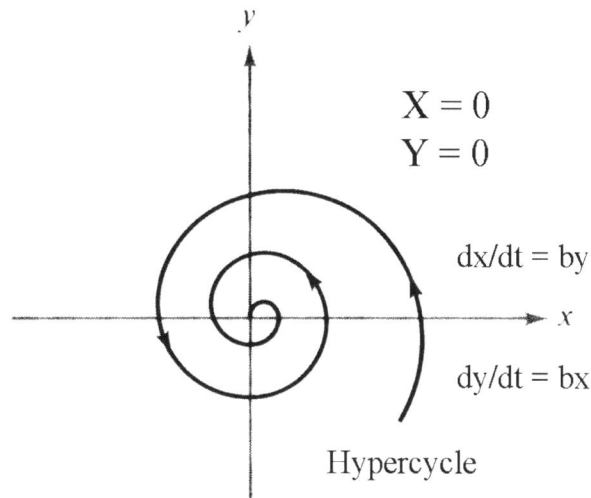

Also, rather than the idea that there is a continuous flow (at certain hours), the Hui hypothesis shows a distinct amount of energy emitted at times, presumably from the pulse generator of an organ or pathogen. Bio-chemical evidence supports this theory. Since external Qigong influences changes to the dimensions of the circle, internal Qigong presumably could also influence it as well through synchronization of the organism through various techniques of practice. In science Prigogine proposes similar diagrams supported by mathematical acceleration formulas in a non-equilibrium natural state. Traditional Chinese Medicine proposes a movement toward equilibrium or stability. In the Hui hypothesis there is very little equilibrium, in fact the basis is a non-equilibrium state, much like a biological organism experiences – changes in hot/cold, high/low atmospheric pressure, humidity/dryness, light/dark, invasion of pathogens, old age, growth, psychic disturbances, trauma, water balance in the body, cosmic bombardment, and modern electro-magnetic fluid fluctuation by electro-magnetic pulse generators (refrigerators, power tools, cell phones, etc.). Internally generated field energy projected outside the body through distant healing, by self-care practices, would support this theory. A quantum amount of purple energy (in Phase1.3) directed by a person's will can be directed outside the body for healing.

CHAPTER TEN
CLINICAL EXPERIENCES
WITH THE O-RING TEST

ITALIAN PHYSICIAN ADRINAO BORGNA'S M.D., EXPERIENCE WITH BDORT

In 1989 I started using the BDOR-test in my practice in Italy having attended a few seminars with Dr. Omura.

The first case was a man that had suffered with chronic sinus problems and was having a flare-up. I had samples of several antibiotics and using the BDORT I found that Erythromycin would have been the most effective. I explained to the patient that besides the antibiotic I also wanted to use the method described by Omura as "drug uptake enhancer" by using a small needle "Pionex" (that resembles a small thumb tack) held in place by a small piece of tape on Stomach 36 (one of the major acupuncture points) and have the patient press on it 30 minutes after the ingestion of the antibiotic.

The sinus problems disappeared within two days but the patient started to feel dizzy, light headed, and faint every time he stood up. The measurement of his blood pressure in a sitting and standing position revealed "orthostatic hypotension." This subject had been on medications for essential hypertension for 5 years. I was a bit surprised but I remembered Dr. Omura talking about infection of "*heart representation area*" in the medulla oblongata as a cause of essential hypertension. I instructed the patient to stop the B/P medications and all the symptoms disappeared. Remarkably his blood pressure monitored daily by the patient himself stayed within normal ranges.

The second case regarded a young woman whom had been classified as "*hysterical*" by another physician. She presented with a general sense of chronic fatigue, malaise and depression. She complained of a metallic taste in her mouth and decreased sense of smell.

The BDOR test indicated lead poisoning. Upon further questioning she told me that her husband was an avid hunter and they often ate the game he hunted. They especially liked small birds called "tordi" (Thrush in English), very good tasting birds, but often the small lead pellets were embedded in their meat and ingested. Further blood-work revealed high levels of lead.

I was very impressed with the accuracy of the method and after attending more seminars I used it more and more until I started testing for cancer, having purchased samples of the cancer markers (Tromboxane B2, Integrine and Oncogen-C-fos) Dr. Omura used during one of the seminars. I was soon caught in a dilemma, because I started to find that a great percentage of people tested positive for those cancer markers but the majority of these people were affected only by minor ailments.

The very first person I told he had cancer got very upset with me because he underwent a complete standard medical examination and CT scan that did not show any tumor or cancer in his body. I knew from Dr. Omura's teaching that BDOR test is extremely sensitive and can detect cancer at the very early stages when it is too small to be detected even by the most sophisticated modern imaging technology.

The dilemma was: shall I tell a patient he has cancer, based on this method, knowing that the potential psychological impact could cause a tremendous stress? Or shall I not tell and put the patient at risk of a more advanced stage of cancer? Appendix I is the Informed Consent Form that we mentioned earlier as a practical step to help overcome the legal aspect of it, although I am still not sure about the ethical and moral position to take. I now use the BDOR Test for food and drug testing and for finding EMF but for the most part I stay away from testing for cancer unless I know the patient well and I feel comfortable with her/his reactions.

In today's practice I find myself using the BDORT to test the innumerable supplements people take. For the most part the BDORT shows me that people spend an incredible amount of money in supplements that have no effect and many are actually harmful. I found very troubling that most of the multivitamins show a negative BDORT response. Of course it is very difficult to pinpoint the component that is causing the negative response given the long list of elements present in the multivitamins but in my experience they are not useful.

Another very useful aspect of the BDORT is its use in the ergonomic assessment of a workspace or the evaluation of some patient environment. It is remarkable how easy it is to identify an electromagnetic field or any other kind of disturbance that can affect a patient. I often examine the bedroom and the workspace of the patients with chronic problems. Especially with chronic pain it is very useful to be able to examine a patient at the location where he/she feels that the pain is at its worst. I first examine the space using the BORT and then I use EMF finders (Tri-Field) not to be influenced by the instrument findings. If the instrument is able to detect a field, the BDORT is always able to confirm the disturbance, however many times the BDORT show abnormalities even though the instrument is not detecting anything. In the latter case I generally trust the BORT over the instrument.

I have been using the BDORT for almost 20 years now and I am still amazed by the accuracy of the method. I do not use it with every patient but when in doubt I rely on it.

ISRAELI NERI KEDEM'S EXPERIENCE WITH THE BDORT

Neri Kedem is a specialist in the use of the O-Ring to evaluate diagnostic and treatment patterns. Kedem teaches shiatsu and other techniques of Japanese Medicine including Sotai, the use of magnets, and the O-ring. Using the O-ring and a Manaka Ion-Pumping Cord found a good and easy way to determine accurately the right point or combination of points that relate(s) to the reactive abdominal point for effective treatment. His particular interest has been finding the connections between the many different forms of treatments and their diagnostic patterns by using and developing simple and easy methods of diagnosis.

I am a native of Israel and work in a clinic in a community setting (the kibbutz where I live) in the southern part of Israel. Previously, I practiced in Tel Aviv and established a shiatsu department in one of the biggest schools of alternative medicine in Israel. I lectured there for nine years. I was one of a group of practitioners that helped establish the first public health maintenance clinic of its kind in the country.

I began my study of Oriental Medicine in 1990 at the Ohashi Shiatsu Institute in New York. I returned to Israel in 1995. I then studied and practiced a variety of therapeutic techniques. This included Japanese Acupuncture therapies, mainly kiiko Matsumoto's style, magnets, Sotai assisted movement therapy, and primarily Dr Omura's diagnostic method, the Bi-Digital O-ring Test (BDORT), which I first read about in the books by Yoshiho Manaka MD and Kiiko Matsumoto (modern Japanese master acupuncturists). Since then I have developed a unique therapeutic approach in which I combine the BDORT as the main diagnostic tool integrated with the other treatment techniques I have learned.

Most of my patients who come to the clinic do so with orthopedic problems or aches and pains. However, I found they were not all purely mechanical problems or orthopedic in nature but involve impaired blood flow, immune system factors, hormonal imbalance, digestive system pathologies and other factors.

Until I started working with the BDORT, my feeling as a therapist was one of uncertainty. It was difficult to diagnose a patient's state, mainly due to the difference in the various methods I employed, especially due to the many different diagnostic 'maps' of the back and abdomen area that are the main diagnostic tools of these modes of therapy. In conjunction with the other diagnostic methods I use, the BDORT is without doubt the most efficient, the most precise and the easiest diagnostic tool I have found to date. It enables me to find the source of the problems in my patients without resorting to conventional test paraphernalia, to supernatural senses, intuition, or any other form of guessing.

I now define my clinic as "third generation medicine," especially for the ability to make very accurate diagnoses using the BDORT, equal to or even better and more precisely than conventional diagnostic methods. Combined with the techniques of diagnosis and therapy of Oriental medicine that I also use, this allows me to better understand the state of my patients, and to succeed in solving their problems safely and promptly, and with a minimum of side effects. I'm pleased with this, as are my patients.

My main contribution to the field beyond using Omura's simple and efficient diagnostic technique is in finding the right acupuncture point using the Omura O-Ring to treat and understand their effects by locating their relationship and connection to the physiological systems and functions of the human body combining Western medicine and the Meridian system of Oriental medicine. Thus the connection between the two methods, oriental and orthodox western medicine, is strengthened. In Israel, alternative medicine is well regarded, but people sometimes have difficulty trusting and following my recommendations. Trust is an important issue with patients. I believe my approach helps to reach a common language – the language and terms of therapy, which I think will enhance the level of therapy itself.

One illustrative example of important information I found working with the BDORT, is the connection between Fire Points of Classical Chinese Medicine and the thymus gland of the immune system. In Oriental medicine these fire points are connected energetically to the 'Heart' and the 'Small Intestine'"

An example of a new diagnostic/treatment method I helped developed is called 'Point Resonance Technique' is described below:

POINT RESONANCE TECHNIQUE
EQUIPMENT

1. One Ion Pumping Cord (IPC). The renowned Japanese acupuncturist, Yoshio Manaka MD, designed the IPC. The IPC is a copper wire with a germanium diode at one end and clips at both ends to attach to needles or electrodes. The black clip is '-' [denoted negative polarity] and the red clip is '+' [denoted positive polarity]. The device's name comes from the inventor's conceptual model of 'ionic current' flowing from the black clip to the red clip against the direction of normal electron flow and diode connection, and which formed part of the protocols invented for the device. (Many practitioners internationally have documented that they have been able to reproduce Dr Manaka's results.) If an IPC is not available, then a conducting lead can be used. But the IPC has the advantage of being directional.
2. Silver Spike Point (SSP) silver-plated brass electrodes if available or any other conducting electrode.

METHOD

(1).The basic method and arrangement for the BDORT is established through a correct match of fingers. The initial O-Ring that is tested is called the 'Control O-Ring'.
(2). A point/area that has clear pathological pressure pain and/or tests positively with the basic BDORT Dysfunction Localization Method is located in the abdomen or on any part of the body. The point/area is considered a reflex point of a functional change of some kind.

(3). The BDORT is used to determine which organ-meridian(s) are creating the pathology detected on the point/area in (2) by using histological organ tissues, slides or photomicrographs of organ tissue which detect electromagnetic resonance between two identical substances.

(4). A SSP is placed on the reflex point using surgical tape (if an SSP is not available the technique can still be easily used - see Note B below). The black clip of the IPC is attached to the SSP and is stationary during the procedure.

(5). The red clip is attached to a second SSP that is moved and touched sequentially from point to point along the meridian of the organ that was identified as contributing to the reflex point located and identified in (2) & (3). At each acupoint, it is also held in place with surgical tape.

(6). At each point that the red clip is touched to and held to with tape, the Control O-Ring is tested. If there is a positive BDORT (complete weakening of the O-Ring) then this indicates that there is a resonance phenomenon between the two points on the body, meaning that the point that the red clip is connected is a reflex point and is a good treatment point.

(7). The identified treatment is stimulated with shiatsu, a needle, or moxibustion. Most often this will reduce or completely take away the pain on the reflex point and/or significantly improve the BDORT on this point.

METHOD TWO
EXTRA EQUIPMENT

A brass or metal probe is substitute for the IPC.

All preparations are identical to Method One.

(8) The patient or the BDORT assistant holds the probe that is softly touched to the reflex point. At the same time an SSP or some other mechanical stimulator is moved and touched sequentially from point to point along the meridian of the organ that was identified as contributing to the reflex point. At each point it is held in place with surgical tape.

(9) At each point along the meridian that the SSP is attached to, the Control O-Ring of the patient or of the assistant if the indirect method is used is tested. When the appropriate point along the meridian is mechanically stimulated by any means, the Control O-Ring of the patient or assistant is strengthened and will not open. This clearly indicates that the point that is being stimulated along the meridian relates to the organ reflex point and will be an effective treatment point for that reflex point. If more than one effective point is found by this method, the BDORT analogue scale can be used to differentiate the best treatment point - which is the point that results in the strengthening of the most O-Rings of the patient or assistant.

NOTES

These methods are not limited to testing standard Traditional Chinese Medicine (TCM) acupoints to a reactive abdominal point or a point elsewhere on the body identified as pathological or pain point. The red clip of the IPC can be placed on any point close to or away from a TCM acupoint.

If electrodes are not available, a small piece of aluminium foil can be taped on the reflex point and the black clip can be attached to the foil. The red clip can be held to the points being checked - by the patient with their hand that is not making the O-Ring, by holding the non-conducting cover of the red clip instead of taping it to the point each time. For greater accuracy, a brass (or other conducting) probe can be inserted into the red clip and touched to the distal points. If the patient touches a conducting part of the IPC near the red clip a short circuit will result and the technique will fail. The black clip can also be taped directly to the reflex point if electrodes are not available.

If there is a positive BDORT on many points on the same meridian that the red clip of the IPC is attached to, this is considered to indicate a definite correspondence between the reflex point and the meridian that is being tested. In this case, in order to identify the best point or a reduced number of points on the meridian that will have the maximum effect on the reflex point, the recommended procedure is to measure and compare using a BDORT analogue scale the resonance of several points on the meridian to the reflex point. The one or two points that have the maximum resonance with the reflex point should be chosen as points for treatment. The analogue scale is achieved by starting testing the Control O-Ring and then sequentially testing the O-Rings made by the subject with their thumb and consecutively stronger fingers than those used to form the Control O-Ring. If the Control O-Ring was formed with the index finger and the thumb, or if this O-Ring is reached and tests positively (i.e. opens) at any time during the testing, then the analogue scale is continued by means of the examiner pulling this strongest O-Ring with O-Rings formed with their thumb and consecutively weaker fingers.

Sometimes one reflex point (on the abdomen) will be found to relate simultaneously to more than one organ-meridian system, any combination is possible. (This is an explanation why combination point treatments often are effective in Japanese style acupuncture for 'clearing' abdominal reflexes). In such cases, two or three points anywhere on the body (on different meridians) can be treated simultaneously with two or three IPCs, shiatsu, needles or moxibustion.

Reversing the connections of the IPC from treatment point to reflex point for a few seconds to a few minutes is also often very effective. Most often this will reduce or completely take away the pain on the reflex point and/or significantly improve the BDORT on this point. And to my clinical experience, it also has the ability to mobilize heavy metals for secretion to the urinary bladder and treat viral and bacteria infections. In these cases the pathogenic area is covered with aluminium foil paper or needled at the approximate middle point with shallow insertion. In stubborn and difficult cases one treatment with this method is not sufficient and repeated treatments will be necessary. The best way to confirm the successful result is by using the appropriate Reference Control Substance. This method alone is not sufficient in severe cases and other forms of therapy need to be combined. For example, the right medication with the right dosage at the time of the treatment. Usually when there is viral and bacteria infections the Fire Point of the TCM meridian of the infected organ or meridian has the greatest degree of resonance to that organ.

AUSTRALIAN RICHARD MALTER'S EXPERIENCE WITH THE BDORT

I am an Australian clinical practitioner using primarily the Bi-Digital O-ring (BDORT) in treating a broad range of clinical cases as a primary diagnostic from orthopedic post-operative pain to orthodox medically diagnosed cancer cases.

I have worked under mentorships resulting in clinical research with a background in shiatsu and acupuncture. I became interested in the BDORT through the published works of Yoshio Manaka, M.D., studying about its basic method and application for diagnosis and evaluation of acupuncture. My colleagues in clinical practise are a medical doctor, a naturopath and a physiotherapist, with the latter two assisting with the BDORT using the indirect method elsewhere explained in this work [1].

I began my investigations of acupuncture and shiatsu diagnosis with the Traditional Medicine of East Asia diagnostic method of palpating for abnormal tenderness or 'pressure pain' at specific organ-related reflexes at locations directly superficial to the position of internal organs and also distal to them on the front and back of the body. Through this investigation I have developed a new diagnostic methodology. Its main feature is the ability to objectively and reproducibly identify and test, in 'real-time', causal inter-organ relations. That is, for any patient with multiple organs involved in their illness or clinical presentations, we have been able to identify the organ that first triggered and continued to be the main influence on the development of the pathology of the other organs involved. Using this system we have been able to make an underlying diagnosis and then give effective treatment in many different cases often when standard and standardly practiced Oriental medicine have failed. By effectively treating the organ that is responsible for the underlying pathology, there have been many clinical successes even in (chronic) difficult cases (undiagnosed) by orthodox medicine. This system is only possible using the BDORT.

I like palpation diagnosis because it is one of the few methods that allows clear and objective, instant feedback about the efficacy of acupuncture (AP) point stimulation on target organs (explained below), rather than relying on popular theoretical and anecdotal considerations. Palpation diagnosis of this kind (explained further below) also contrasts with the common confusion regarding the 'de qi' needle sensation often relied upon by traditional acupunctures that is a neurological phenomenon that does not necessarily give useful information about the effect on target organs is of AP point stimulation. However, I wanted to understand the subject better than I had found in the existing literature, and also to fill in some of the many obvious gaps in theory and clinical practice on the subject in both Traditional Chinese Medicine (TCM) textbooks and in modern Japanese-origin AP treatises.

In AP and some meridian shiatsu systems, an Organ Representation Point (ORP), termed a mu and shu point in TCM (often translated as 'alarm points'), is a small area on the surface of the body where an existing pathology of an internal organ can be detected by palpation. Some Japanese-origin AP systems theoretically relate many additional, distal reflex points or areas ('distal ORP's), in the abdomen and elsewhere on the front and back of the body, to internal organs for diagnosis. The clearest palpable indication of pathology on an accurately located ORP of an organ or distal ORP is palpation pressure evoked pain, 'pressure pain' (PP). In some Japanese-origin AP systems, disappearance ('clearing') of this PP from an ORP or distal ORP as a result of stimulation of AP points during a treatment session is also used as an objective and a reliable indicator of successful treatment. An example of a clinically useful ORP that often has PP is the TCM location for detecting liver pathology, Liver-14 (LV-14) AP point that clinically includes a transverse area approximately 4cm long centering on LV-14 in the 6th intercostal space approximately on the mammilary line. Sharp PP at this location (differentiated clearly from normal tenderness in the intercostal space) is usually a clear sign of liver pathology of some kind and degree. However there are many more that have not been documented clearly in traditional literature.

As discussed earlier, the BDORT resonance phenomenon between two identical substances can discover pathological organs, directly or indirectly. In our study, proximal and distal PP reflexes were found by comprehensive physical examination of 50 subjects. From experience, these reflexes were considered to relate to varied clinical symptoms of unidentified internal organ pathology rather than being of underlying musculoskeletal origin. Palpation was made as deep as necessary and appropriate. For example, palpation of the ovaries was often made 5-6cm deep into the body depending on the amount of fatty tissue lying immediately above them. Locations with clear, strong reflexive PP were marked. The BDORT resonance phenomenon between two identical substances was then used to identify which internal organ(s) where contributing to PP at each localized area. Sometimes the organ(s) identified were not anatomically near to the PP reflex. Accurate ORPs of other organs that we had not found any related PP either superficial to them or distally were then also located directly above them with the BDORT and marked. Overall, reflexes identified included the liver, pancreas, kidneys, adrenal glands, stomach, ovaries, gallbladder, intestines, etc.

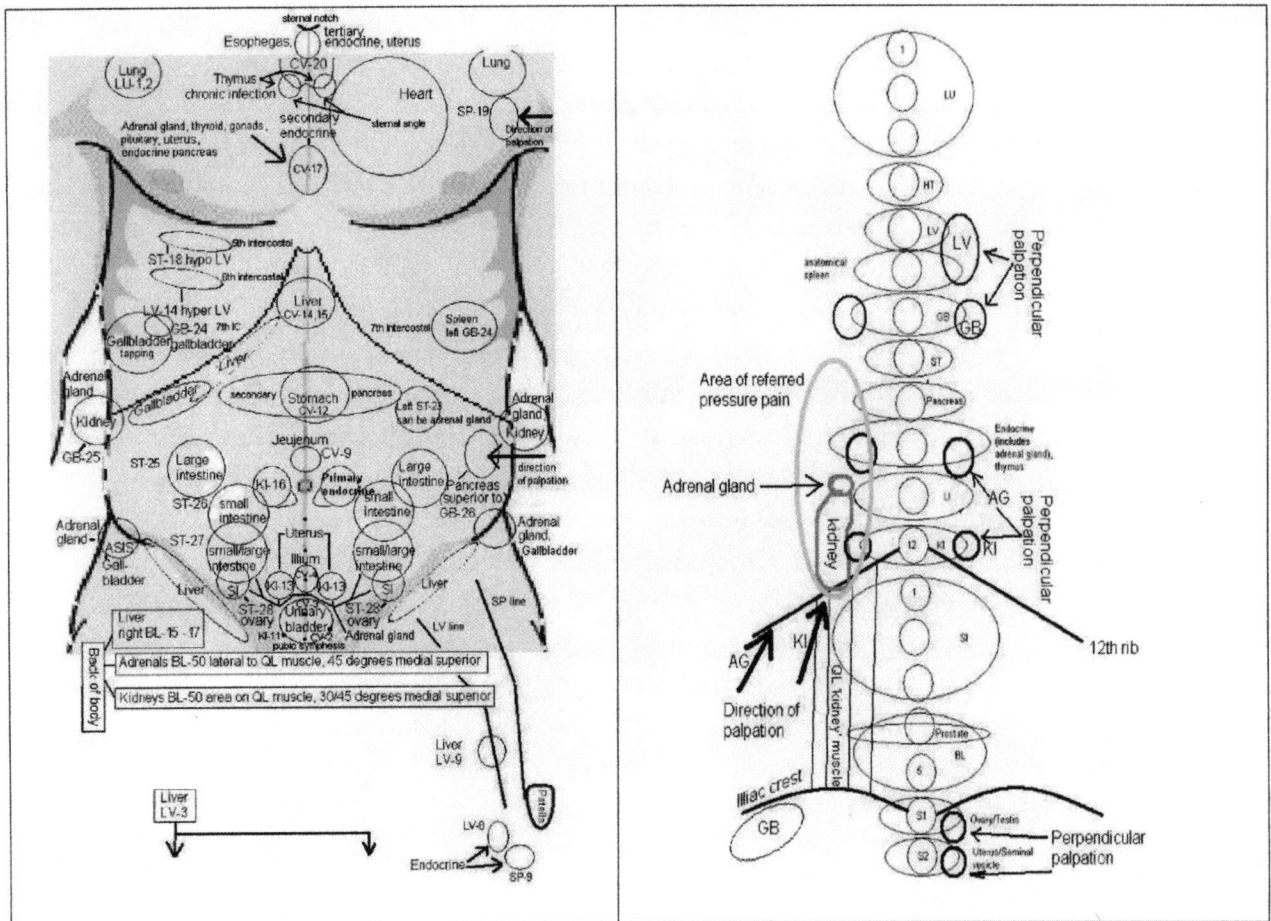

***Figure 1: Anterior and posterior palpation diagnosis reflexes
identified with BDORT resonance phenomenon between two identical substances***

With this simple to apply approach we improved on palpation diagnosis in terms of accuracy and scope from the standard teaching syllabus of TCM courses and some well known Japanese-origin AP systems (see Fig 1). We continued to analyze and evaluate palpation diagnosis in detail. This was done by using the BDORT resonance phenomenon between two identical substances to detect and measure a number of biochemical and non-organic substances in each organ for which we had found ORPs and distal ORPs (see Fig 2 and below for non-organic influences). It was found that palpation diagnosis for PP often but not always correlated with BDORT diagnosis. Palpation diagnosis was found to have great clinical usefulness when corrected and improved as described. However, it was also found that often there is significant pathology of an organ that can easily be detected by measuring the same BDORT parameters (given in Fig 2) when there is no detectable related PP from that organ. This is a critical finding regarding palpation diagnosis of this kind as it shows that it is not foolproof. Furthermore, because of the speed of the BDORT, we could measure these parameters in many organs effectively simultaneously to find out, via AP point stimulation, how any one organ affected one or more organs. In many instances, we were also able to find out how one or more organs created or affected a specific symptom. For example, using this methodology, we have found repeatedly that a major or primary underlying causal pathological dynamic in the many cases of spleen, thyroid, colon, pancreas, prostate, uterus, rectal vein, portal vein, vertebral and carotid artery problems, is actually related to a liver pathology. This simple finding helped to solve many cases that were treated unsuccessfully for many years.

Biochemical parameter	Description All measurements are Bi-Digital O-Ring Test Units (BDORTU)
1. Function	Basic BDORT (+6 ~ -6)
2. Telomere (synthesized base code TTAGGG)	i) Significantly lower telomere (approximately from >100ng lower to up to 500ng lower) than normal cell telomere: the organ is considered to be relatively hypo-pathological. Above the bicep is used as a standard location for measurement of normal cell telomere. ii) Significantly higher telomere (approximately from >100ng higher to 900ng higher) in comparison to normal cell telomere: the organ is considered to be relatively hyper-pathological
3. Circulatory disturbance	ThromboxaneB2 (TXB2) was the control reference substance. Normal parameter value: ≤1ng.
4. Neurotransmitter Acetylcholine (ACh)	1mg was the normal parameter value

Figure 2

The following points are the main findings of our study. The last point (2) gives an actual overview of the new diagnostic methodology already mentioned.

1) Organic and non-organic Influences on Organs (systems) and Limitations of AP Treatment

Significant organ pathology, which is often 'subclinical' and does not show up in standard tests, can be detected and evaluated with the BDORT by measuring a number of biochemical and non-organic chemical parameters at several locations inside the BDORT imaged outline of the organ where there is no super-positioning with another organ using the BDORT resonance phenomenon between two identical substances. Organ-specific telomere measurement is a very useful marker for hypo and hyper activity of an organ compared to the measurement of normal cell telomere usually taken on the upper arm above the biceps. ThromboxaneB2 indicates a microcirculatory disturbance such as restricted blood supply to an area and possible spasticity. Acetylcholine, a key neurotransmitter, is often dramatically reduced in pathological organs. Since this study we also always measure organ-specific L-homocysteine as a necessary and very useful vascular inflammation marker. Other frequently found highly significant parameters inside organs (sometimes contributing to PP at an ORP or distal ORP) are non-organic toxins such as mercury, asbestos, lead, aluminium, arsenic, chromium and cadmium, in any combination. All of these factors can lead to and entrench micro-organism invasion. (Intracellular) viral and bacterial infections also sometimes contribute to organ related PP. Only the BDORT can non-invasively detect and measure these intracellular non organic toxins and infections with high accuracy. In instances when a pathological organ has one or more PP reflexes, often on a distal ORP of that organ, the direct influence of the adrenal glands was found also to be a very significant and frequent causal factor of the PP and related pathology. The adrenal glands may be pathological or reacting normally to other pathological dynamics in the body. In addition, in instances of non-organic toxicity and/or infections, we found that the beneficial effect of appropriate AP point(s) stimulation only maintained a short time and we could measure over a few minutes the reversal of the BDORT parameters to pathological ranges. In such instances the Selective Drug Uptake Enhancement Method [OMURA Y, 1996-] is the effective solution.

A single ORP and/or (distal ORPs) are not always sufficient to diagnose an organ accurately or comprehensively. For example, in a large organ such as the liver, most of the organ may be functioning normally with normal range BDORT parameters (and gives no PP), while a smaller surrounding area has multiple, intra-cellular viral and bacterial infections and also high intra-cellular mercury toxicity which can easily be detected and measured with the BDORT. The relatively small pathological area is enough to contribute to a very wide variety of clinical symptoms elsewhere. Palpation diagnosis in such cases is not very accurate.

2) Testing Causal Dynamic Inter-Organ Relations in Pathology

Amongst the parameters detected with the BDORT, specific organ telomere (compared to normal cell telomere) is an extremely useful indicator of both hyper and hypo conditions of organs. It is also one of the key parameters that allow the simple and quick 'real time' discovery of the causal relationship of one pathological organ on another pathological organ on an individual patient basis. The methodology is very simple and logical. BDORT parameters (discussed above) are measured in a number of organs that might be involved in the clinical or symptomatic presentations from a basic knowledge of medical physiology. An appropriate AP point of one organ is determined and stimulated non-invasively with nanocurrent from 30 seconds to 2 minutes. We use a number of simple methods to objectively select the (best) appropriate AP point(s) in any instance – some of which we have developed ourselves [10]. These AP point selection methods are practical and do not rely on theoretical considerations. BDORT parameters are then immediately re-measured in the same organs as before. Patterns of causal inter-organ relationships are then seen vividly and conclusively. A chief example of a key inter-organ dynamic that we utilize daily in our clinic is the liver-thyroid relation. In our clinical experience, of the possible many factors contributing to any thyroid pathology, the factor that comprises approximately 80% of all the causal influences on the thyroid pathology is an underlying liver pathology. The remaining 15-20% of all the causal influences on any thyroid pathology is adrenal gland pathology. Gonad pathology is the possibly remaining 5%. This is demonstrated in 'reversed-time-order' by the fact that in the majority of cases appropriate AP point stimulation of the liver immediately normalizes the telomere of the thyroid gland lobes. These relationships can only be demonstrated and measured (in 'real time') with the BDORT. Though the liver-thyroid relationship is common knowledge and has been investigated in very great detail in modern medical science, a review of the existing medical literature shows that this relationship is almost completely ignored for therapeutic purposes. Medication, irradiation or surgical removal is the orthodox medical approaches for thyroid pathology.

This new methodology has solved the problems of many patients who were otherwise destined to lifetimes of unnecessary medication, operations, and ever-increasing ill health.

In cases where standard test results, such as of a Liver Function Test, have previously detected these pathologies, success of our treatments has also been confirmed by improved results of the same standard tests when repeated, at a rate of approximately 90%. In many other cases, only the BDORT discovered the pathologies, which were 'sub-clinical' and explained what were otherwise (often chronic) undiagnosed conditions. This methodology is entirely objective and reproducible and so it can be applied very widely. From clinical experience, I am convinced it can stop use, and dependency on enormous amounts of unnecessary pharmaceutical drugs in any given western population.

A PHILOSOPHY OF MEDICINE FROM CLINICAL PRACTICE

There is also a philosophy (of medicine) involved and promoted by this methodology, that daily use of the BDORT has shown and impressed upon me, which I think is very important and that this method serves as an example to illustrate a more general principle: an energetic systems approach is far closer to nature than the chemical-mechanistic reductionist one that is currently the method of orthodox medicine.

Our study therefore also contextualized and put into fuller perspective a traditional medicine practice and its concepts, and it extended from them further to improve the understanding and clinical practice of diagnosis of internal organs.

APPENDIX I

I, _____ hereby authorize the use of the Bi-Digital 0-Ring Test" upon myself (or my ward, _____), by Dr. _____. I understand that this test is considered experimental. The "Bi-Digital O-Ring Test" was explained as a simple non-invasive, safe and quick new diagnostic method gradually developed in the US since the early 1970s and has been actively used by some physicians in the USA, Scandinavian countries, Germany, Belgium, Japan, China, Korea and Venezuela since the early 1980s, although it is not known to a majority of physicians and dentists in the USA. Using the Test. It is possible make a systematic diagnosis without knowing the chief complain or history of the patient. It has the following potential adverse psychological impacts, potential adverse effects, and potential benefits:

Potential Adverse Psychological Impacts: 1) Because the high sensitivity of this test, standard laboratory test may fail to confirm the Bi-Digital O-Ring Test results until the disease or symptom further advance. This may give the impression of misdiagnosis and create a psychological conflict for the patient. 2) The results of this test may contain unpleasant or unexpected medical information and some people may suffer mental distress from such information. 3) The selection of a drug and its optimal time duration as suggested by the test may be different from the standard textbook advice; in addition, prolonged use of the drug may be required.

Potential Adverse Effects: Just like any established diagnostic method, there is the possibility of false positive or false negative results for unforeseen reasons.

Potential Beneficial Effects: 1) Because the high sensitivity of this test, many disease can be detected in the very early stages and suitable treatment can be initiated, often at a great saving of time, money, and discomfort. 2) The possibility of microorganisms causing infection can theoretically be detected and localized, and effective treatment for such microorganism can be suggested. 3) The method is completely non-invasive, simple, safe, and painless, unlike most known standard methods. It can be performed almost anywhere as it does not depend on expensive, bulky instruments. 4) Therapeutic effects of any treatment can be quickly and non-invasively evaluated, safely and economically. 5) Without knowing the chief complaint or history of the patient, various abnormalities in different parts of the body can be detected.   6) Imaging of normal and abnormal internal organs can be made non-invasively and safely without exposing the patient to undesirable X-ray, radioactive substances or strong magnetic fields.

7) Neurotransmitters and other substances in the living human can be qualitatively detected non-invasively without taking a biopsy or a blood sample. 8) Through the use of Bi-Digital O-Ring Test, one can select an optimal drug for treatment of a specific problem or affected organ, or detect a toxic food or drug prior to their ingestion.

Because of the highly sensitivity of the O-Ring Test, standard tests results may fail to confirm its results; however the physicians performing the test have the ethical responsibility to inform the patient of possible abnormalities of organs (including the possible existence of cancerous cells and their location), infections that may exist and their possible consequences, as well as possible treatments as indicated by the Bi-Digital O-Ring test results. The physician must leave entirely up to the patient the choice of whether or not to act based on the test results.

The procedure of this test consists of testing muscle strength of the O-Ring formed by the thumb and a pre-selected finger – one that satisfies 3 essential conditions of reproducibility – of the same hand while a minute mechanical force or a very weak beam of light, electric, or magnetic field is applied on the body surface below which the abnormality is suspected. Although I understand that this test is not widely known by the medical community in this country, the method and procedure have been explained to me in details and all my questions have been answered. I therefore authorize

Dr. _____ to make a diagnosis and suggest treatment based on this test. I also authorize the physician doing this procedure to write the findings of the test directly on the body surface and to take a photograph on this as a permanent medical record of this test result. Since this procedure was authorized by my free will, I am free to withdraw at any time from future tests and treatment. I will not blame or sue the physician or the institute or location where such procedure was performed concerning any consequence of the test results or treatment.

Signature of Witness   Signature of Patient / Age/ Date

_____

Witness's Address   Patient's Address

_____

_____

_____

Witness's Phone #   Patient's Phone #

_____

MALTER AND KEDEM REFERENCES

http://bdort.org/BiDigitalORingTestPages/PatentSpecification.htm

Omura. Y. Acupuncture Training Course Supplement. International College of Acupuncture & Electro-Therapeutics, pp39-47, 2006.

http://www.bdort-prt.net/PalpationDiagnosis.htm

Matsumoto K. Kiiko Matsumoto's Clinical Strategies Vol.1, pp4-6, Kiiko Matsumoto International, 2004.

Manaka Y. Chasing the Dragon's Tail: The Theory and Practice of Acupuncture in the Work of Yoshio Manaka, pp141-144, 118-119. Paradigm Publications, 1995.

Shinnick P. "The Application Of The Bi-Digital O-Ring Imaging Test To Toxic Organ Meridians And Clinical Medicine". American Journal of Medical Acupuncture, Vol. 14: #3, pp29-35, 2003.

Omura Y. "New simple early diagnostic methods using Omura's "Bi-Digital O-Ring Dysfunction Localization Method" and acupuncture organ representation points, and their applications to the "drug & food compatibility test" for individual organs and to auricular diagnosis of internal organs-part I". AEJ.IJ, 6(4), pp239-54, 1981.

Omura Y. "Re-evaluation of the classical acupuncture concept of meridians in Oriental medicine by the new method of detecting meridian-like network connected to internal organs using Bi-Digital O-Ring Test". AEJ.IJ. 11(3-4), pp219-31, 1986.

Omura Y. "Meridian-like networks of internal organs, corresponding to traditional Chinese 12 main meridians and their acupuncture points as detected by the Bi-Digital O-Ring Test imaging method: search for the corresponding internal organ of Western medicine for each meridian-Part I". AEJ.IJ, 12(1), pp53-70, 1987.

Cao, Xiao-Ding. "Scientific [Neuroanatomical and Neurochemical) Basis of Acupuncture and Acupuncture Treatment-Review of Historical Developments in the People's Republic of China". Presented at 22nd International Symposium of Acupuncture and Electro-therapeutics, New York, USA 2006.

Kedem N, Malter R. "The Bi-Digital O-Ring Test - Point Resonance Techniques: Simple and Accurate Ways of Diagnosis and Treatment in Organ-Meridian Oriental Medicine". North American Journal of Oriental Medicine, Vol.13 #38, pp10-15, 2006.

Omura Y. "Accurate Localization of Organ Representation Areas of the Tongue, using the Bi-Digital O-Ring Test: its clinical application, and re-evaluation of classical Oriental Tongue Diagnosis - Part 1". AEJ. IJ, 16, pp27-43, 1991.

KITADE T, Toshikatsu K. "Clinical Investigation of the Location of Meridians and Acupoints by Means of Bi-Digital O-Ring Test(I): Heart Meridian in Normal Subjects and Patients with Atrial Fibrillation". Japanese Journal of Ryodoraku Medicine, Vol. 46:3, pp152-163, 2001.

Voll R. "Twenty Years of Electro acupuncture diagnosis in Germany. A Progress Report". American Journal of Acupuncture, Vol. 3(1), pp5-17, 1975.

Omura Y. "Basic electrical parameters for safe and effective electro-therapeutics [electro-acupuncture, TES, TENMS (or TEMS), TENS and electro-magnetic field stimulation with or without drug field] for pain, neuromuscular skeletal problems, and circulatory disturbances". AEJ.IJ, 12(3-4), pp201-25, 1987.

Omura Y. "Treatment of acute or chronic severe, intractable pain and other intractable medical problems associated with unrecognized viral or bacterial infection: Part I". AEJ.IJ, 15(1), pp51-69, 1990.

Omura Y, Losco BM, Omura AK, Takeshige C, Hisamitsu T, Shimotsuura Y, Yamamoto S, Ishikawa H, Muteki T, Nakajima H, et al. "Common factors contributing to intractable pain and medical problems with insufficient drug uptake in areas to be treated, and their pathogenesis and treatment: Part I. Combined use of medication with acupuncture, (+) Qi gong energy-stored material, soft laser or electrical stimulation". AEJ.IJ, 17(2), pp107-148, 1992.

Malter R, Loader A, Tyrrell H. "Normal Thyroid Function And Hormone Range Depend On Narrow Range Of Optimal Liver Parameters". 24th Annual International Symposium on Acupuncture & Electro-Therapeutics and Related Fields, New York, USA, 2008.

Malik R, Hodgson H. "The relationship between the thyroid gland and the liver". Q J Med 2002; 95: pp559-569.

ENDNOTES

CHAPTER ONE

1.   Shinnick, P and Omura,Y. "Difference in the Location of Finger Placement on the Radial Artery for Pulse Diagnosis in the Orient; and, 15th to 18th Century Occidental Rare Books on Pulse Diagnosis." Acupuncture & Electro-therapeutics Research, the International Journal. Vol. 10: 309 -324, 1985.

2.   Shinnick, P. Freed, S. Blumenthal, C, & Omura, Y. The Heart. The Heart Disease Research Foundation 50 Court Street Brooklyn, NY 11201. (p. 14,17)1987

3.   Shinnick, P. "Modern Acupuncture Techniques: An Introduction to the Basic Technique and Theory of Omura's Bi-Digital O-Ring Test." American Journal of Acupuncture. Vol. 24: 2/3, 1996

4.   Shinnick, P. "The Application of the Bi-Digital O-Ring Imaging Test to Toxic Organ Meridians and Clinical Medicine." Medical Acupuncture. Vol. 14: 3. 30-35 2003.

5.   Losco, M. "Suggestions for Performing the Bi-Digital O-Ring Test." AER,IJ. Vol. 16: 1/2. 53-64 1991

6.   Omura, Y. "Bases Biofisicas y Bioquimicas. (Electro Acupuncture & Manual Acupuncture: Biophysical and Biochemical Bases) Electro Acupuncture y Acupunctural Manual: EDAD S.A., Marcaibo, Venezuela", 1984.

7.   Omura, Y. "Practice of Bi-Digital O-Ring Test". Ido-No-Nihon-Sha, Tokyo, Japan, 1986. (In Japanese)

8.   Omura, Y. Acupuncture Medicine, "Its Historical and Clinical Background." Japan Publications, Inc. Tokyo, Japan, 1982.

8a   Omura, Y. "Relation between transmembrance action potential of single cardiac cells and their corresponding surface electrograms in vivo and in vitro and related electro-mechanical phenomena." Transaction of the NY Academy of Science. Series, ll, Vol. 32: No. 8. 874-940. Dec 1970.

9.   Omura, Y. "Critical evaluation of the measurement of "tingling threshold" " pain threshold" and "pain tolerance" by electrical stimulation." AER, IJ, Vol. 1: 3/4, 161-236, 1977

10.   Omura, Y. "Pain threshold measurement before and after acupuncture: Controversial results of radiant heat method and electrical method, and the roles of ACTH-like substances and endorphins", AER, IJ, Vol. 3: 1/2, 49-96, 1978

11.   Omura, Y. "Effects of an electrical field and its polarity on an abnormal part of the body or organ representation point associated with diseased internal organs, and its influence on the Bi-Digital O-Ring Test (simple non-invasive dysfunction localization method) & drug compatibility test-Part 1." AER,IJ, Vol. 7: 4, 209-246, 1982.

12.   Omura, Y. "Applied kinesiology using the acupuncture meridian concept: Critical evaluation of its potential as the simple non-invasive means of diagnosis, and compatibility test of food and drugs- part 1", AEJ. IJ, Vol. 4: 3/4,165-183,1979.

13.   Omura, Y. "Simple and quick non-invasive evaluation of circulatory condition of cerebral arteries by clinical application of the "Bi-Digital O-Ring Test." AER,IJ,Vol. 10: 3, 139-161, 1977.

14.   Omura, Y. "The Bi-Digital O-Ring Test: Critical evaluation of its abnormal responses with laboratory test including " blood pressure & blood flow method", "blood chemistry", etc., and " neurological method." AEJ. IJ, Vol. 8: 1, 37-43, 1983

15.   Omura, Y. "Non-invasive circulatory evaluation and Electro-Acupuncture and TES treatment of disease difficult to treat in Western medicine: 1) abnormal brain circulation and blood pressure: cephalic hypertension or cephalic hypotension syndromes and their related conditions-insomnia, blindness due to macular degeneration and retinitis pigmentosa, and some psychiatric problems; 2) severe lower extremity circulatory disturbances, with intractable pain, intermittent claudicatio, ulceration and/ or severe diabetic neuropathy," AEJ. IJ, Vol. 8: 3/4, 177-256, 1983

16.   Omura, Y. "New simple early diagnostic method using Omura's "Bi-Digital O-Ring Test dysfunction localization method" and organ representation points, and the applications to the " drug and food compatibility test" for individual organs and to auricular diagnosis of internal organs." AEJ. IJ, Vol. 6: 4, 239-254, (p. 254)1981.

17.   Omura, Y. "Acupuncture (with possible roles of serotonin and melatonin) and related unorthodox methods of diagnosis and treatment: Non-invasive spheno-palatine ganglinonic block, abrasion of naso-pharyngeal mucosa, and applied kinesiology."AER,IJ, Vol. 4: 2, 69-90, 1979.

18.   Omura, Y. Part 1, AEJ, IJ, Vol. 4: ¾, 165-184, 1979.

19.   Omura, Y. "Effects of an electrical field and its polarity on an abnormal part of the body or organ representation point associated with a diseased internal organ, and its influence on the Bi-Digital O-Ring Test (simple, non-invasive dysfunction localization method) drug compatibility test-Part 1." AEJ, IJ, Vol. 7: 4, 209-246, 1982.

20.   Omura, Y. "A new, simple, non-invasive imaging technique of internal organs and various cancer tissue using extended principles of the " Bi-Digital-O-Ring Test" without using expensive imaging instruments or exposing patients to any undesirable radiation Part 1". AEJ, IJ, Vol. 10: 4, 1985.

21.   Omura, Y. "Bi-digital-O-ring test Molecular Identification and Localization Method' and its Application in Imaging of internal Organs and Malignant Tumors as Well as Identification and Localization of Neurotransmitters and Micro-Organisms Part 1", AEJ, IJ, Vol. 11: 2, 65-100, 1986

22.   Omura, Y. "Meridian-like networks of internal organs, corresponding to traditional Chinese 12 main meridians and their acupuncture points as detected by the "Bi-Digital O-Ring Test Imaging Method": Search for the corresponding internal organ of Western Medicine for each meridian." AEJ, IJ, Vol. 12: 1, 53-70. (p. 59)1987.

23.   Omura, Y. "*Stress & Immunity and the effect of stimulation of deep personal nerve at St. 36 on ventricular arrhythmia, heat disease & sudden death.* New simple accurate and inexpensive imaging technique of internal organs and cancer tissue by a clinical application of "Bi-Digital O-Ring Test" and clinical significance of newly discovered networks of thymus gland in cancer treatment*", AEJ, IJ, Vol. 10: 1/2, 1-12 1985.

24.   Omura, Y., Losco, M., Omura, A.K., Takeshige, C., Hisamitsus, S., Nakajima, H., Soejima, K., Yamamoto, S., Ishikaima, H., Kagoshima, T., Watari, N., Shimotsura, Y., Matsubara, T. "Bi-Directional transmission of molecular information by photon or electron beams passing in the close vicinity of specific molecules, and its clinical and basic research application: 1) diagnosis of humans or animal patients without any direct contact; 2) light microscopic and electron microscopic localization of neuro-transmitters, heavy metals, Oncogen C-fos (AB2), etc. of intra-cellular fine structures of normal and abnormal single cells using light or electro-microscopic Indirect Bi-Digital O-Ring Test." AER, IJ. Vol. 17: 1. 29-46, 1992.

CHAPTER TWO

25.   Omura, Y. "Electro-magnetic resonance phenomenon as a possible mechanism related to the Bi-Digital O-Ring Test, molecular identification and localization method." AEJ, IJ, Vol. 11: 2, 127- 145, 1986

26.   Takeshige's theory was recorded in presentation at the Omura seminars from 1988-1990.

27.   Weigle, W. "Self/non-self recognition by T and B lymphocytes and their role in auto-immune phenomena. "Arth Rhrum," Vol. 24: 8, 1044-1053, 1981

28.   Simon, F. "Induced specific immunological unresponsiveness and conditioned behavior reflexes in functional isomorphism." AEJ, IJ, Vol. 44: 275-283, 1988

CHAPTER FOUR

29.   Omura, Y. "*Re-evaluation of the classical acupuncture concept of meridian in Oriental medicine by the new method of detecting meridian-like networks connected to internal organs using the Bi-Digital O-Ring Test.*" AEJ, IJ, Vol. 11: 3/4, 219-231, 1986

30.   Omura, Y. "*Connections found between each meridian (heart, stomach, triple burner, etc.) & organ representation area of corresponding internal neurotransmitters and hormones unique to each meridian and corresponding acupuncture point & internal organ after acupuncture, electrical stimulation,*

mechanical stimulation (including shiatsu), soft laser stimulation or Qigong." AEJ, IJ, Vol. 14: 2 155-186, (p. 173, 174)1989

31.   Omura, Y. "Editorial: (2) New Simple Accurate and inexpensive Imaging Technique of Internal Organs and Cancer Tissue by a Clinical Application of "Bi-Digital O-Ring Test" and Clinical Significance of Newly Discovered Network of Thymus Gland in Cancer Treatment." AER,IJ, Vol. 10: 1/2, 4-5. (p. 5)1985

31A.   Omura, Y. "The Bi-digital O-Ring Test Molecular Identification and Localization Method and his application in imaging of the internal organs and malignant tumors as well as identification and localization of neurotransmitters and micro-organisms - Part 1" AER,IJ, Vol. 11: No 2 pp.66-89 (p. 81, 7A, B and C)1986.

32.   Omura, Y. "Accurate Localization of Organ Representation Areas of the Tongue, Using the Bi-Digital O-Ring Test: Its Clinical Application, and Re-evaluation of Classical Oriental Tongue Diagnosis—Part I." AEJ, IJ, Vol. 16: 1/2, 27-44, (p. 34)1991

33.   Omura, Y. Organ Representation Areas of the Hand Localization by the Bi-Digital O-Ring Test. IDO-NO-NIPPON-SHA Shinjuku-ku TOKYO 160   JAPAN

CHAPTER SIX

34.   Omura, Y. Simple and Quick Non-Invasive Evaluation of Circulation condition of cerebral arteries by clinical application of the "Bi-Digital O-Ring Test." AER,IJ. Vol. 10: 139-161, (p. 146)1985

35.   Omura, Y. "Interrelationships Between the Heart and Central Nervous System: Localization of Neuro-Transmitters and Imaging of their Associated Nuclei, Including the Raphe Nuclei & the Locus Coeruleus, as well as the Imaging of the Heart and its Representation Areas in Slices of the Human Central Nervous System Using the "Bi-Digital O-Ring Test" Imaging method." AER,IJ, Vol. 12: 1/2, 139-164 (p. 156)1987

36.   Omura, Y. "Connections found between each meridian (heart, stomach, triple burner, etc.) & organ representation area of corresponding internal organs in each side of the cerebral cortex; release of common neurotransmitters and hormones unique to each meridian and corresponding acupuncture point & internal organ after acupuncture, electrical stimulation, mechanical stimulation (including shiatsu), soft laser stimulation or Qi Gong." AEJ, IJ, Vol. 14: 2 155-186, (p. 165)1989

37.   Omura, Y. "Abstracts of the 3rd International Symposium on Acupuncture and Electro-Therapeutics: Simple method of imaging of internal organs and their corresponding meridian-like network and non-invasive localization of neuro-transmitters in slices of brain tissue and in living human brain. " AEJ, IJ, Vol. 12: 3&4 245-292 1987.

38.   Omura, Y. Transmission of molecular Information through Electro-Magnetic Waves with Different Frequencies and its Application to Non-Invasive Diagnosis of Patients as well as Detection from Patient's X-Ray Film of Visible and Not Visible Medical Information: Part I, AER, IJ, Vol. 19: 39-64, 1994

39.   Omura, Y. "Bi- directional transmission of molecular information by photon or electron beams passing in the close vicinity of specific molecules, and its clinical and basic research applications: 1) diagnosis of humans or animal patients without any direct contact; 2) light microscopic and electron microscopic localization of neurotransmitters, heavy metals, Oncogen C-fos (AB2), etc. of intracellular fine structures of normal and abnormal single cells using light or electro-microscopic Indirect Bi-Digital O-Ring Test." AER, IJ, Vol. 17: 1, 29-46, 1992

39A.   Omura, Y. "Treatment of Acute or Chronic severe Intractable Pain and other Intractable Medical Problems Associated with Unrecognized Viralor Bacterial Infection: Part I" AER,IJ, Vol. 15: pp. 51-69 (p.60)1990

40.   Omura, Y. "The Bi-Digital O-Ring Test: Critical evaluation of its abnormal responses with laboratory test including 'blood pressure & blood flow method', 'blood chemistry', etc., and 'neurological method'." AER,IJ, Vol. 8: 1, 37-43, 1983

41.   Omura, Y. "Storing of Qi gong Energy in Various Materials and Drugs (Qi Ionization): Its clinical Application for Treatment of Pain, Circulatory Disturbances, Bacterial or Viral Infections, Heavy Metal Deposits, and Related Intractable Medical Problems by Selectively Enhancing Circulation and Drug Uptake" AER, IJ, Vol. 15: 137-157, 1990

42.   Omura, Y. "Unique changes found on the Qi Gong (Chi Gong) Master's and patient's body during Qi Gong treatment: Their relation to certain meridians & acupuncture points and the re-creation of The rapeutic Qi Gong states by children and adults." AER,IJ, Vol. 14: pp. 61-89 1989

43.   Omura, Y., Losco, M., "Electro-Magnetic fields in the home environment (color TV, computer monitor, microwave oven, cellular phone, etc.) as potential contributing factors for the induction of Oncogen C-fos Ab1, Oncogen C-fosAb2, Integrin alfa5 b1 and the development of cancer, as well as effects of microwave on amino acid composition of food and living human brain" AER,IJ, Vol. 18: 33-73 1993

44.   Omura, Y., Losco, M., Omura, A.K., Takeshige, C., Hisamitsus, S., Nakajima, H., Soejima, K., Yamamoto, S., Ishikaima, H., Kagoshima, T., Watari, N., Shimotsura, Y., Matsubara, T. "Bi-Directional transmission of molecular information by photon or electron beams passing in the close vicinity of specific molecules, and its clinical and basic research application: 1) diagnosis of humans or animal patients without any direct contact; 2) light microscopic and electron microscopic localization of neuro-transmitters, heavy metals, Oncogen C-fos (AB2), etc. of intra-cellular fine structures of normal and abnormal single cells using light or electro-microscopic Indirect Bi-Digital O-Ring Test." In AER, IJ, Vol. 17: 1 29-46, 1992

45.   Omura, Y., Shimotsura Y., Ooki M., Nogucht T. "Estimation of the Amount of Telomere Molecules in Different Human Age Groups and the Telomere Increasing Effect of Acupuncture and Shiatsu on St.36, Using Synthesized Basic Units of the Human Telomere Molecules as Reference Control Substances for the Bi-Digital O-Ring Test Resonance Phenomenon" AEJ, IJ, Vol. 23: 185-206, 1998

46.   Omura, Y. "Transmission of Molecular Information through Electro-magnetic Waves with different Frequencies and Is Application to Non –Invasive Diagnosis of Patients as well as Detection from Patient's X-ray Film of visible and Not Visible Medical Information: Part I." AER,IJ, Vol. 19: 1 1994

47.   Ozerkan, K. "*The Effects of Smiling or Crying Facial Expressions on Grip Strength, Measured With a Hand Dynamometer and the Bi-Digital O-Ring Test*" AER,IJ, Vol. 26: pp. 171-186, 2001

48.   Alwasa, S., Neves, L.B., Lopes, A.C., "*The Importance of Bi-Digital O-Ring Test in the Treatment of Multiple Hepatic Abscesses- A Case Study*" AER,IJ, Vol. 28: pp. 201-206, 2003

49.   Asou, T., Hayashi, T., Jitsuik, I., Muneshige, H., Nagatomi, A., Kaseguma, E., "A Patient with MRSA Infection to Prosthesis of Femoral Head Diagnosed Non-Invasively Using Bi-Digital O-Ring Test: A Clinical Case Report" AER,IJ, Vol. 28: pp. 69-72, 2003

50.   Omura, Y., Shimotsuura, Y., Ohki, M., "2 Minute Non-Invasive Screening for Cardio-Vascular Diseases: Relative Limitation of C-Reactive Protein Compared with More Sensitive L-Homocystine as Cardio-Vascular Risk Factors; Safe and Effective Treatment Using the Selective Drug Uptake Enhancement Method." AEJ, IJ, Vol. 28: 35-68, 2003

CHAPTER NINE

51.   Omura, Y. et al. AETR,IJ, Vol. 14: No. 2 p. 173.

52.   Omura, AETR,IJ, Vol. 13: No. 4 p.157

53.   Omura, AER,IJ, Vol. 4: No. 2, p.175

54.   Prigogine, Ilya "Being to Becoming: Time and Complexity in the Physical Science." W.H. Freeman and Company. San Francisco p.146, 1980

55.   Prigogine. p.107